Therapeutic Relationships with Offenders

Forensic Focus

This series, edited by Gwen Adshead, takes the field of Forensic Psychotherapy as its focal point, offering a forum for the presentation of theoretical and clinical issues. It embraces such influential neighbouring disciplines as language, law, literature, criminology, ethics and philosophy, as well as psychiatry and psychology, its established progenitors. Gwen Adshead is Consultant Forensic Psychotherapist and Lecturer in Forensic Psychotherapy at Broadmoor Hospital.

in the same series

Sexual Offending and Mental Health
Multidisciplinary Management in the Community
Edited by Julia Houston and Sarah Galloway
Foreword by Dawn Fisher
ISBN 978 1 84310 550 3

Personality Disorder
The Definitive Reader
Edited by Gwen Adshead and Caroline Jacob
ISBN 978 1 84310 640 1

Therapeutic Interventions for Forensic Mental Health Nurses
Edited by Alyson Kettles, Phil Woods and Mick Collins
ISBN 978 1 85302 949 3

Working Therapeutically with Women in Secure Mental Health Settings
Edited by Nikki Jeffcote and Tessa Watson
Foreword by Jenni Murray
ISBN 978 1 84310 218 2

Boys Who Have Abused
Psychoanalytic Psychotherapy with Victim/Perpetrators of Sexual Abuse
John Woods
Foreword by Arnon Bentovim with a contribution from Anne Alvarez
ISBN 978 1 84310 093 5

A Matter of Security
The Application of Attachment Theory to Forensic Psychiatry and Psychotherapy
Edited by Friedemann Pfäfflin and Gwen Adshead
ISBN 978 1 84310 177 2

Forensic Focus 30

Therapeutic Relationships with Offenders

An Introduction to the Psychodynamics of Forensic Mental Health Nursing

Edited by Anne Aiyegbusi and Jenifer Clarke-Moore

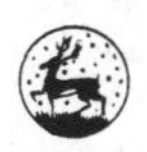

Jessica Kingsley Publishers
London and Philadelphia

The authors and publishers are grateful to the proprietors listed below for permission to quote the following material:
Extract from 'The Second Coming' by William Butler Yeats, copyright © W. B. Yeats 1919, reprinted in W. B. Yeats Selected Poems (2000), London: Penguin, p.124. Reproduced by permission of A P Watt Ltd on behalf of Gráinne Yeats.
Extract from 'From Pain to Violence: The Traumatic Roots of Destructiveness' by Felicity de Zulueta, 2006. Copyright © John Wiley & Sons Limited. Reproduced with permission.

First published in 2009
by Jessica Kingsley Publishers
116 Pentonville Road
London N1 9JB, UK
and
400 Market Street, Suite 400
Philadelphia, PA 19106, USA

www.jkp.com

Library of Congress Cataloging in Publication Data

Therapeutic relationships with offenders : an introduction to the psychodynamics of forensic mental health nursing / edited by Anne Aiyegbusi and Jenifer Clarke-Moore.

p. ; cm.

Includes bibliographical references.

ISBN 978-1-84310-949-5 (pb : alk. paper)

1. Forensic psychiatric nursing. 2. Nurse and patient. I. Aiyegbusi, Anne. II. Clarke-Moore, Jenifer.

[DNLM: 1. Forensic Psychiatry. 2. Psychiatric Nursing. 3. Countertransference (Psychology) 4. Nurse-Patient Relations. 5. Nurses--psychology. 6. Prisoners--psychology. WY 170 T398 2009]

RA1155.T479 2009

614'.15--dc22

2008029082

British Library Cataloguing in Publication Data

A CIP catalogue record for this book is available from the British Library

ISBN 978 1 84310 949 5

Printed and bound in Great Britain by
MPG Books, Limited, Cornwall

Contents

This book is dedicated to Dr Estela V. Welldon who first made psychodynamic work with offenders accessible to us as nurses and whose vision, creativity and clinical wisdom has served as an ongoing inspiration.

Introduction

Anne Aiyegbusi

The world of forensic mental health nursing is often difficult to describe to those who have not experienced prolonged clinical contact with patients at the therapeutic interface of secure services first hand. Even then, the characteristic, intense emotional phenomena that tend to arise out of interpersonal relationships with patients and colleagues are not easy to articulate. Yet, for those of us who consider our professional identity to be one of 'forensic mental health nurse', it seems important to find a way to put words to what appears to occupy a large component of our working lives. More importantly, if we can develop a framework for making sense of the way our work makes us feel, we will be in a better position to harness our energy and enthusiasm in the service of supporting forensic patients towards a pathway to recovery. Of course, forensic patients are supported through services with or without a theoretical framework for articulating nurses' emotional experiences. However, this frequently occurs in the context of significant struggle. For patients, this struggle is often characterized by difficulty communicating what their needs are and for nurses this struggle is often characterized by feeling emotionally overwhelmed by their task of providing containing, therapeutic relationships for patients whose interpersonal needs are not clear to them.

The aim of this text is to clarify some important interpersonal and emotional needs that underpin forensic patients' presentations within the clinical environment, in a way that is accessible to nurses. While the text is by no means an attempt to address the many facets of theory, practice, legislation and security that make up the whole of the forensic nurse's task, it does attempt to provide a detailed insight into one of them. That is the nurse–patient relationship which is an aspect of practice that distinguishes us from our multiprofessional colleagues. The nurse–patient relationship is at the core of relational security but it takes place within a balanced matrix which also includes systems of physical and procedural security. While not focusing on procedural and physical systems of security, the text does not aim to underplay their importance either. However, no apology is made for highlighting relational aspects. This is because there is a relative dearth of literature available to guide forensic mental health nurses in their challenging relational task. Also, it is felt that emphasizing this component of the nursing role will be both validating and supportive of those struggling with the emotional impact of their work at the clinical interface of secure services.

A psychodynamic approach has been taken because the authors of this text have found it to be a useful way of capturing the richness of clinical nursing experience in forensic services. A psychodynamic framework also provides a way to work effectively within challenging forensic services offering a language for the complex emotional and behavioural phenomena that can often feel puzzling or indeed overwhelming. While emphasizing reflectivity and the need to think even when under extreme pressure to act, the psychodynamic model also offers a framework for informing therapeutic action. The key is in understanding the difference between action that perpetuates the patient's difficulties and action that supports the patient to discontinue damaging patterns of relating. The authors of this collection of chapters have largely referred to their extensive clinical experience within a range of forensic mental health nursing services and the related field of services for people with severe personality disorders.

While this text does not attempt to provide the last word in incorporating a psychodynamic perspective to the care of offenders, it is hoped that it might go some way toward offering a first word in terms of a way for forensic mental health nurses to work effectively with complex interpersonal phenomena. It is also hoped that this text will inspire nurses to open up an avenue of therapeutic endeavour informed by an awareness of unconscious processes. These intangible forces bring about a powerful influence within clinical environments, in relationships between patients and professionals and at an organizational level, yet relatively little attention is paid to them in the course of day-to-day practice within forensic services. In taking account of unconscious processes, as will be evident in the chapters that comprise this text, there is a need for professionals as well as patients to develop self-awareness with regard to motivations for finding ourselves working in forensic mental health services. Likewise, emphasis is placed upon mobilizing the functional part of patients as well as the part that experiences difficulty or mediates risk behaviours. This is sometimes difficult to achieve within environments that are dominated by systems of control. However, doing so within forensic contexts represents a challenge to be met by nurses. The final point to make is that what is being advocated in this text is that a psychodynamic model, when integrated with other theoretical frameworks, can strengthen clinical nursing practice. The key message is one of integration and with that in mind it is hoped, too, that further enquiry into the emotional impact of working as a nurse in forensic mental health services will be reflected in future research studies.

In Chapter 1, Anne Aiyegbusi explains the value of integrating a psychodynamic perspective into forensic mental health nursing practice. A series of case examples convey the ways in which nurses can find themselves failing to grasp their patients' needs and are unable to 'hear' their communications. Anne focuses on containment of unthinkable emotional states as a starting point for establishing the nurse–patient relationship with people detained in forensic services. Clinical nursing processes and practices required to maintain safe, boundaried, therapeutic relationships are explored in this chapter and it is argued that containment of toxic emotional states better enables the nurse to fulfil their role of supporting and facilitating the recovery of patients detained in forensic mental health services. In Chapter 2, Malcolm Kay discusses Winnicott's theory of hate in the counter-transference, recognizing that it is often impossible or taboo for nurses to think about their hateful feelings towards the patient. It is suggested that forensic nurses cannot avoid hating their patients at times. It is also suggested that acknowledging and understanding such feelings will make a significant and positive difference to the way nurses are able to deliver care and treatment to patients. In Chapter 3 Gillian Tuck discusses forensic systems and organizational dynamics, drawing on ideas developed at the Tavistock Centre, a tradition which integrates open systems theory with psychoanalytic concepts. In doing so, light is shed on some of the complex dynamics that become manifest within secure organizations. This is followed by Chapter 4 which explores the particular organizational defences that are likely to emerge in forensic institutions. By applying the principles identified in Isobel Menzies' landmark paper on social defence systems in a general nursing service to the forensic mental health nursing context, Amanda Lowdell and Gwen Adshead clarify the particularly intense and often non-thinking atmosphere of the forensic mental health service.

In Chapter 5, Anne Aiyegbusi explores the dynamics of difference, describing the psychodynamic processes that are central to understanding human beings' propensity to discriminate against one another, sometimes in hateful, hurtful ways. Why forensic mental health services may be prone to creating environments characterized by painful interpersonal relating that usually involve various forms of attacking difference is explored in this chapter. Nursing processes and practices that aim to work thoughtfully and effectively with the dynamics of difference are also described.

Chapters 6, 7 and 8 focus on intense, destructive psychopathology, including that which may be regarded as dynamically psychotic. In Chapter 6, Valerie Brown explores some of the psychodynamic concepts that have helped her to understand the emotional environment of the secure mental health setting she works in. Valerie explains how an understanding of unconscious processes which are derived from the Kleinian model of the paranoid-schizoid position supports her clinical nursing practice. In Chapter 7, Stephen Mackie considers some aspects that are involved in weekly ongoing staff support groups in forensic secure settings. Stephen describes their usefulness and the form of support they can provide as well as exploring aspects that can make them difficult for both the members of the group and the facilitator. Stephen explains that many different and diverse issues arise in ward reflective practice groups but perhaps the most difficult to explore is that of destructiveness and murderousness, aspects that inevitably percolate throughout a secure forensic service as a result of its containment of violent, psychotic offenders. In Chapter 8 Sarita Bose applies Bion's psychodynamic concept of psychological containment to the provision of a structured daily programme of activities for a detained forensic psychiatric population. Containment is emphasized in relation to its usefulness within the admission facilities in any forensic psychiatric hospital.

Chapters 9, 10 and 11 focus on the role of the nurse in different services for people who have personality disorders. In Chapter 9, Christopher Scanlon and John Adlam focus on the persistent threat to psychic survival faced both by nurses and patients in forensic settings, how these threats become manifest in the dynamic interplay between nurses, others within the multidisciplinary team and those mentally disordered offender patients who are perceived to be dangerous. In Chapter 10, Neil Gordon explores the impacts upon nurses of working with personality disordered men in a high security psychiatric hospital environment. Neil begins by discussing the psycho-political nature of these environments and the ambivalent attitudes society holds towards those who are cared for in these settings. This is followed by a brief discussion of the relationship between theory and practice. In the final part of Chapter 10 Neil focuses on the relational world of the forensic mental health nurse illustrating through a fictitious clinical supervision narrative how this ambivalence can emerge in the mind and the behaviour of those who inhabit this context. In Chapter 11, Rebecca Neeld and Tom Clarke consider the structural elements of the therapeutic community and how these serve to organize, contain and aid the therapeutic relationship. Following a brief overview of the clinical setting, Rebecca and Tom explore aspects of the therapeutic community from the patient's and then the nurse's perspective. Fictional vignettes drawn from clinical practice are used to illuminate processes.

Chapters 12, 13, 14 and 15 focus on the care of women in secure services. In Chapter 12, Suzanne McMillan and Anne Aiyegbusi describe how they developed a nursing workforce able to intervene effectively with the complex care-seeking communications engaged in by women patients detained in secure mental health settings. They will discuss how patients and ward-based nurses in their different ways can be understood as crying out for care in the face of overwhelming anxiety and distress associated with unprocessed traumatic phenomenology. In Chapter 13 Katie Downes discusses how the mutual suspicion that is so often a central part of the relationship between patients and nurses in secure settings can be used effectively within a culture of enquiry to support patients whose complex needs have the potential to unbalance the nurse. In Chapter 14 Jenifer Clarke-Moore and Miranda Barber explore the challenges forensic nurses face when working with women in secure services and the need to develop an integrated model of nursing care based on the development of secure base behaviour. Jenifer and Miranda draw from attachment theory and describe how a clinical model derived from this theoretical framework can provide effective care and treatment for women within a medium secure setting. In Chapter 15, Joanne Roberts and Jenifer Clarke-Moore describe how they first met each other as service user and charge nurse within a medium secure unit. They reflect upon their journey together as they have moved through different roles over a period of 15 years. This chapter tells Joanne and Jenifer's story up until the point that they work together to develop a new forensic service as user consultant and consultant nurse. The aim of this chapter is to provide an insight into forensic mental health nursing from the user perspective as well as the nurse's. Joanne and Jenifer emphasize that we have a lot to learn from one another.

Finally, in Chapter 16, Maria McMillan describes some aspects of working as a forensic community mental health nurse within a Youth Offending Team. Maria explains the challenge of working as a nurse in this setting in terms of the adolescent offender's unconscious wish for such a figure being complicated by his developmental need to separate from his parents, who are inevitably parents with whom the adolescent has a very chaotic and damaged attachment. Maria illustrates through case examples how the forensic nurse's therapeutic aim is to ensure that the adolescent's painful reality should not be avoided or denied, but be felt, tolerated and then, one hopes, understood.

CHAPTER 1

The Nurse–Patient Relationship with Offenders: Containing the Unthinkable to Promote Recovery

Anne Aiyegbusi

INTRODUCTION

In this chapter I will explain the value of integrating a psychodynamic perspective into forensic mental health nursing practice. The material within the chapter is largely derived from extensive clinical work in the field of forensic nursing. In keeping with the rest of this book, the chapter aims to apply a framework to interpersonal relating with patients including manifest emotional experiences that are well known to forensic nurses. The intention is for nurses working in the forensic field to have greater awareness of the containing function of their interpersonal work, recognizing that uncomfortable feelings are part of it and that these feelings can be put to effective clinical use providing good enough support and reflective space is embedded within the structure of services. This will provide nurses with an opportunity to process those difficult feelings that their patients cannot. Furthermore, I hope to argue that a psychodynamic approach to working with forensic patients will support nurses to apply the recovery principles of valuing patients' aims, promoting hope and optimism with regard to change, social inclusion and working in partnership with patients that are described in the chief nursing officer's review of mental health nursing (Department of Health 2006).

The chapter will begin by presenting a number of fictional case examples that aim to reflect some of the difficult aspects of human relating that nurses are tasked with managing professionally and therapeutically when engaging with forensic patients. Each case example will be followed by a discussion, describing some of the dynamics that might underpin the relational scenarios and, also, how an 'ear' to the unconscious and the presence of containing structures might have enabled nurses to better support the patients and themselves.

CASE EXAMPLES

Case example 1

John is a 38-year-old man who has been detained in a secure hospital for many years. His index offence involved abduction, sexual assault and manslaughter of a young boy. He has a diagnosis of severe antisocial personality disorder. For several weeks John had been observing a new student nurse on his ward. This student nurse, a young man in his early twenties, is struggling to find his feet in this new environment and has been subject to mild teasing by his experienced colleagues, including his mentor and some of the other patients, because of his apparent slowness. He has also been publicly on the receiving end of some practical jokes. These pranks and jokes seem to make the student nurse all the more awkward in his role.

John, who is very familiar with the workings of the ward, begins to offer himself as a source of help to the student nurse, showing him where to find things on the ward and reminding him of various aspects of the daily routine. The student nurse finds John to be very helpful at a time when he does not feel able to turn to his colleagues for support and is thinking that he is not suitable for his career. He finds himself wondering why John is in a secure hospital at all. The student nurse has requested to be placed in John's nursing team because he feels they have begun to develop a therapeutic relationship. John, who has hitherto not been known for his engagement with professionals, has no difficulty asking for one-to-one sessions with the student nurse. The student nurse gladly provides the one-to-one sessions though he does not write them up fully in John's case notes, nor does he receive supervision for them from his mentor.

In a routine room search, a small number of benzodiazepines are found secreted in John's toiletries. John is not prescribed any medication. He says that the student nurse has given these drugs to him. At the student nurse's disciplinary hearing, he admits that John had complained of severe, debilitating anxiety in their one-to-one sessions. John had said that because of his diagnosis, nurses and doctors did not believe that he could also experience distress and that he was being treated as though he were less than human. John had been relentless in his complaints about the 'system' and how he was treated within it. The student nurse had felt that he owed John because of how supportive he had been during a time when the student nurse had felt vulnerable. The student nurse had brought in some of his own mother's benzodiazepines and given them to John in the hope that he might feel relief from his distress. John had asked the student nurse to do this after the student nurse had discussed his mother's emotional problems and treatment in response to John's interest in his family background.

Discussion of case example 1

Case example one demonstrates how the relationship between an inexperienced member of nursing staff and a forensic patient can become corrupted. John might be considered predatory in his 'grooming' of a young student nurse who was seemingly alienated from his professional group. In actual fact, he had managed to isolate the victim of his index offence in a similar manner. The student nurse did become unconsciously identified with John's victim in that he was overpowered by the more dominant personality, looking to John for support at a time when he felt vulnerable in his professional role. Through a lack of understanding about the psychopathology of a man like John, failing to maintain professional boundaries and not receiving supervision or adequate mentoring, the student nurse was not able to function in the role of an associate nurse. John was easily able to pull him out of his role and take advantage. The student nurse, in a professional sense, abused the patient by giving him un-prescribed medication which had been smuggled into the hospital from home and so also breached hospital security systems as well as his professional code. However, he did so because the patient had convinced him that by doing as John wanted, he would be helping him, a victim of a brutalizing system. In identification with what John reported, the student nurse also felt somewhat brutalized during his introduction to the hospital.

Case example 1 raises questions about the therapeutic milieu of the ward John was residing on. The lack of a model for organizing the nurse–patient relationship with a patient group that included men as dangerous as John meant that the student nurse had no way of understanding what he needed to do, in an interpersonal sense, to at least maintain safety for himself and John. The defensive relationships between staff included the high use of practical jokes which served to divert attention from the deadly serious nature of their patients' psychopathologies. Practical jokes, though traditionally seen as part of a system of institutional humour, strongly communicate a failure to attend to professional boundaries and a contempt for vulnerability, possibly reflecting aspects of sado-masochism originating within the patient group in the first instance but acted out by the staff group. Supervision may have alerted a more experienced nurse to the unhealthy nature of the relationship between the student nurse and John at an early stage while also identifying how John was able to split the student nurse off from his colleagues, but because this was not embedded within the ward structure, the student nurse was left to become isolated from his colleagues and became naively drawn into a collusive, pathological relationship with a dangerous patient. This case example also raises questions about the student nurse's vulnerability and how this was responded to by his colleagues and by John who may have been unconsciously working together, re-enacting a drama from John's internal world.

If, in a dynamic sense, for every victim–perpetrator dyad there is also a third party unconsciously colluding by turning a blind eye, then the ward team in this case example must surely represent the carer who failed to protect. As a learner on the ward, the student was vulnerable but this was compounded by personal characteristics that rather marked him out as being particularly needy of support and the input of his more experienced colleagues. It seems that established ward staff had no time for that vulnerability and as well as attacking it directly through practical jokes and the like, they also seemed unable to keep the student safe within this placement. He was exposed to a dangerous patient without having the experience, skills or knowledge about how to practise safely. As such, it could be argued that from the perspective of a re-enactment, the student, John and the established ward staff were all drawn into re-creating the detail of John's index offence which in dynamic terms mirrored abuse experienced in his childhood. The failure of all professionals to contain John's psychopathology can also be seen in this case example. If John was unconsciously seeking containment through his coercion of the student nurse, he did not receive it until the room search revealed his store of drugs. At this point John was in effect able to draw attention to the unsafe practices on the ward that had enabled him to undermine security systems and engage in his own abusive behaviour within the hospital setting. As is often the case with the dynamics of forensic care, more than one scenario may be operating at any given time with the roles of victim, perpetrator and non-protecting carer ever changing.

Case example 2

Richard is a 27-year-old man who grew up in care. He has been detained in a medium secure unit for one year. He has a diagnosis of paranoid schizophrenia and his index offence involved affray and threatening members of the public with a knife in response to auditory hallucinations whereby he heard voices telling him shoppers were devils in disguise. Richard responded well to medication but was left feeling lethargic by it. Richard knows that he will soon be discharged from the medium secure unit and is very worried about how he will live the rest of his life with a severe mental illness.

Richard's primary nurse is a young man of similar age who has recently married. Richard feels he has a good relationship with his primary nurse who is kind to him and sorts out any day-to-day problems he might have. However, Richard has noticed that the primary nurse does not seem to want to talk in any depth about anything. This is frustrating to Richard who is becoming increasingly anxious about having to live an independent life. Prior to his index offence, he had been living a chaotic existence and had accumulated a lot of debt. He had lost his council flat and was living rough at the time of the offence. Richard is very worried about finding himself in similar circumstances just as he has begun to feel secure and stable within the medium secure unit. The ward social worker has advised Richard many times that he will receive a high level of support for a long time to come but this does not reassure him. As a psychotic patient who is responsive to medication, Richard is not seen by the multidisciplinary team as somebody who requires psychological therapies. He is seen regularly by the ward doctor and their meetings focus on Richard's mental state and his medication regime.

One evening, Richard tries to communicate his anxieties to his primary nurse. He says that he is thinking of coming off his medication. The primary nurse advises him that this would be a big mistake and reminds him of all that he will lose, including the fact that Richard will end up remaining in hospital for much longer. The primary nurse also informs Richard that if he has a relapse of his paranoid schizophrenia as a result of stopping his medication, the chances are that he will never regain his current, high level of functioning. At the next clinical team meeting, Richard is informed by his responsible medical officer that concerns have been raised about his consent to treatment and as a result, a second opinion will be sought so that he can be given medication even if he does withdraw his consent. Richard was also advised that his oral medication was going to be changed to depot to ensure that he takes it.

Discussion of case example 2

In this example a patient's anxieties about survival outside of a secure institution go unnoticed by his primary nurse. The patient was treated for a severe mental illness under the medical model and his underlying human feelings about how to live his life with a condition which he fears will be debilitating appear to be too uncomfortable to be addressed. He does not feel able to put into words how he feels and unconsciously communicates his worries by saying he is thinking about stopping his medication, perhaps to gain the attention of his primary nurse as to how desperate he is feeling. However, his communication is completely missed and instead, increased restrictions under the Mental Health Act (1983) are applied. Furthermore, he is prescribed intramuscular medication. Meanwhile, his anxiety persists.

Often, forensic patients communicate their emotional needs in an indirect way. This may be because they have learned early in life that direct communications of need do not result in the desired care being provided. This pattern of communication may be all the more prevalent in people who have grown up in the care system and who have not had a dedicated, responsive care-giver who is attuned to their needs. When people who have this background are admitted to forensic services, there is a danger that the type of care they received as children will be re-enacted within the secure health care setting.

Richard's primary nurse was a kind man and a dedicated professional but he was unable to attune to Richard's needs and his style of communicating what they are. Richard was not seen as a candidate for psychological therapy which mirrors his childhood experience of never having an individual carer dedicated to his needs. Richard, in his inability to make his needs known in direct, verbal communications, may in the transference have been expecting to be rejected by his primary nurse and so unconsciously attempted to draw attention to the fact he was not feeling safe with regard to pending discharge from the unit by suggesting that he was going to stop his medication. This could have been interpreted in terms of Richard not feeling ready to care for himself and that he had anxieties about being able to stay well. Instead, in the counter-transference, his primary nurse reacted to Richard's pleas, much as the care staff of his childhood had, by resorting to practical rather than emotional support. Had the primary nurse been able to understand that the anxiety Richard projected into him, by saying that he was thinking of stopping his medication, was a reflection of Richard's own anxiety, the latter could have been thought about. Instead, the primary nurse acted on the projected anxiety without giving thought to it and rushed to organize a more controlling, invasive plan of care for Richard.

Richard remains just as anxious about his future and it remains to be seen how he will escalate his communications in an attempt to have his anxieties properly heard and contained. A question raised by case example 2 is why the primary nurse could not 'hear' Richard's communications. Could it be that, as a man of similar age, it was just too painful to engage emotionally with Richard's distress regarding having such a debilitating illness? Whatever underlay the primary nurse's difficulties with engaging with Richard's distress, this case example is a reminder of how important it is to have awareness of our own unconscious motivations for choosing the work we undertake and how we practise within our professional roles.

Case example 3

Julienne is 31 years old and has been detained in a specialist women's secure unit for 18 months. Her index offence was arson. She has a primary psychiatric diagnosis of borderline personality disorder. Julienne has a history of abandonment and abuse in childhood. Her own daughter who is now ten years old was taken into care and adopted as a toddler due to Julienne's inability to care for her. Julienne's index offence involved setting fire to a skip outside the family court where the case for her daughter's adoption was agreed. One of the core areas of need that Julienne presents with on a day-to-day basis is that she makes continual complaints about her treatment in the unit. She complains about all disciplines but is particularly aggrieved with the nursing staff whom she accuses of incompetence and of being 'unfit for purpose'. Julienne frequently makes written complaints to senior members of the management team whereby she describes examples of shoddy practice on behalf of the nurses on her ward. She often makes suggestions about the type of training the nurses require. In the ward community meetings which Julienne usually chairs, she lists all her observations of the nurses from the previous week, describing their shortcomings and what she describes as 'areas of weak practice'. Nurses often feel exposed when Julienne names them personally and they become defensive about their practices, often reminding Julienne that no other patients on the ward complain about them in this way, which is true. Nurses complain amongst themselves about the way Julienne always seems to pick fault with the way they care for the more vulnerable patients on the ward, sometimes when they are engaged in providing direct care. They attribute this behaviour on Julienne's part to her diagnosis of borderline personality disorder.

This pattern of Julienne making complaints and nurses defending themselves, either in interaction with Julienne or as part of complaints or management investigations, has continued throughout Julienne's admission. A mechanism has been put in place to try to ensure all of her complaints are resolved at ward level. However, there is a build-up of resentment amongst many of the nurses who feel demoralized and humiliated by what feels like constant scrutiny into their practice.

Discussion of case example 3

Julienne has a history of failed care in her personal background. She was abandoned by her mother and has a history of childhood abuse. As a mother herself, she was unable to care for her child who was eventually adopted by somebody seen by authorities to be capable of providing proper maternal care. The theme of failed maternal care appears to be central to understanding her internal world. Additionally, her index offence involved setting fire to a skip outside the court where her daughter's adoption was agreed. This indicates the rage Julienne feels about being unable to care for her child and the way this is projected onto authorities. Within the secure unit, this dynamic persists, with Julienne projecting her anger, humiliation and demoralization about being unable to care for her child, and perhaps also the fact that she was not cared for, onto the nurses on her ward. By accusing them of being 'unfit for purpose' she is distancing herself from her own experience of being judged an 'unfit mother'. This of course also links into her distress at having an 'unfit mother' herself. Her efforts to alert managers as to the training needs of nurses could be understood as a communication about her own struggle to be a mother when she had not experienced good enough mothering herself.

If nurses on Julienne's ward had been able to explore the psychodynamics of their relationships with Julienne, they may have been better able to support her with her distress by understanding that the way she was making them feel reflected unresolved, un-thought about distress on her part. In conjunction with colleagues from other disciplines, they might have been able to support her to think about why she was so preoccupied with failed care. As it was, the nurses ended up mirroring Julienne's distress in that they were becoming angry and humiliated because of the continuous accusations. In a way they were providing containment in that while they were preoccupied with what she was doing to them and how they were feeling as a result, Julienne remained somewhat distanced from her core distress. However, this kind of containment has little therapeutic value in the long term because nobody learns anything. Instead, all concerned are maintaining the status quo through a matrix of re-enactments.

INTERPERSONAL WORK IN FORENSIC MENTAL HEALTH SERVICES

Forensic psychotherapists have clarified the challenges associated with close interpersonal work with offenders. Cox (1996) has suggested that professionals working in the forensic field are exposed to particularly intense emotional experiences associated with patients' psychopathologies. In particular, the fact that most patients within forensic services have offended in severe ways brings professionals into close contact with the disturbing fact that the patients have acted out the most primitive of human phantasies such as violence or homicide. As Cox (1996) points out, close interpersonal work with this patient population inevitably puts professionals in touch with primitive parts of themselves which might be experienced as highly disturbing. Defences against emotional experience stirred up by this interpersonal work might, according to Kirtchuk and Haworth (1996), include becoming unconsciously identified with the victim of the patient. Clinical reactions on the part of professionals might include denying the perpetrator part of the patient and engaging only with the pleasant, vulnerable parts or becoming emotionally unavailable for interpersonal work.

Cox (1996) warns that the detail of forensic patients' index offences have the potential to 'whet prurient preoccupations or so horrify that psychological distancing, denial or distraction is the only possible response' (Vol. II, p.444). Temple (1996) also reminds us about the intensity of disturbance encountered in work with forensic patients on account of the large extent to which sado-masochism is often present within interactions and the primitive defences involved. Primitive defences include projection.

Davies (1996) articulates very well the way in which the offender's internal world drama can be acted out by the multiprofessional network. The offender is actually seeking containment but when professionals are unwilling or unable to think about unconscious processes underpinning the criminal act, they are likely to find themselves providing the opposite of what is being sought. That is, rather than being able to provide containment, the multiprofessional network will actually find themselves drawn into a re-enactment. As a result, the offender is prone to escalating their behaviour until containment is finally achieved. As Davies (1996) puts it:

> The view is taken that professionals who deal with offenders are not free agents but potential actors who have been assigned roles in the individual offender's own re-enactment of their internal world drama. The professionals have the choice not to perform but they can only make this choice when they have a good idea of what the role is they are trying to avoid. Until they can work this out they are likely to be drawn into the play, unwittingly and therefore not unwillingly. Because of the latter, if the pressure to play is not anticipated then the professional will believe he is in a role of his choosing. (Vol. II, p.133)

As mentioned previously, nurses experience most of their interpersonal contacts with patients in the open social environment of services where unconscious processes are difficult to monitor and the emotional impact is often experienced as unpredictable. Working in close proximity to groups of patients and to relatively large numbers of professionals complicates the task of monitoring emotional experience and identifying the source of disturbance. As such, it may be difficult for nurses to process their emotional reactions at the time of their occurrence. However, nurses working in the forensic field can learn from what forensic psychotherapists have to say about the psychopathology of offenders and the emotional impact of close interpersonal work.

FORENSIC MENTAL HEALTH NURSING

Nurses working in forensic services are unconsciously invited to process intense, sado-masochistic projections. These sado-masochistic projections reflect the way the offender's internal model for relationships is organized. In turn, the basis for sado-masochistic relating within the forensic population is often an attempt to master trauma whereby vulnerability in some form has been attacked or maltreated in any one of a number of highly distressing ways. If nurses are unable to process these projections, the risk is that they will act upon them, which will interfere with the clinical process and, in particular, will undermine the containing function that nurses have. When professionals working in forensic services become drawn into acting out scenarios, the offender's initial traumas inevitably get re-enacted. Professionals and the wider institutions within which services are located may unconsciously facilitate the re-enactment. In defence of uncomfortable feelings, over-involved or avoidant strategies may be employed.

BOUNDARIES

Freud (1905) recognized that the development of strong, even intense feelings between clinician and patient are an inevitable aspect of therapeutic relationships. Freud was of course referring to the relationship between analyst and patient but the same principle applies to other therapeutic relationships, including the nurse–patient relationship. These strong feelings are largely mediated by unconscious processes and are usually referred to in terms of the transference and counter-transference: that is, feelings stirred up by the therapeutic encounter whereby the patient has feelings toward the clinician which have their origin in an earlier relationship, usually with an early care-giver (transference) and feelings that are stirred up in the clinician which may be best understood as a response to the patient's transference feelings in combination with the clinician's internal world, including motivations for choosing their profession such as unmet needs for care and validation that are projected onto their patients (counter-transference) (Gabbard and Lester 1995). In order to contain these transferences and counter-transferences so that they can be utilized in the service of meeting the therapeutic needs of the patient, rather than for example fueling the acting out of unconscious wishes or re-enacting prior traumatic experiences, boundaries must be maintained. Boundaries in psychotherapeutic practice include meeting the patient at the same time, in the same venue, for the same duration and providing the patient with ample notice of holidays, other breaks in therapy or endings. In private psychotherapeutic practice, fees are another form of boundary maintenance. Additionally, the therapist's training, code of practice, ethical framework, supervision and personal therapy serve in the maintenance of therapeutic boundaries (Brown and Stobart 2008). Brown and Stobart (2008) recognize that it is much more difficult to contain the emotionality of therapeutic encounters and relationships when interpersonal relating occurs in settings and by professionals where the protection afforded by the psychotherapeutic frame is not available. This would be the case for nurses.

As has been described previously in this chapter, transference and counter-transference material present within relationships with forensic patients is particularly potent and is frequently sado-masochistic in nature. The implementation and maintenance of professional, therapeutic boundaries is therefore vital to containing this intense, often difficult and painful emotional material and utilizing it in the service of clinical work. Aiyegbusi (2004) has described the challenge facing forensic mental health nurses in maintaining their professional roles in the face of tremendous interpersonal pressure from patients to act out in ways that are not in keeping with the professional values of nursing. In the light of this pressure to provide a relationship other than that which is professional and therapeutic, it becomes essential that nurses work within a highly boundaried framework. Boundaries in forensic settings include the proper and effective application of the security policies and operational procedures of the organization, working within a structured therapeutic milieu, receiving regular clinical supervision and reflective practice which takes account of transferences and counter-transferences within the nurse–patient relationship, receiving training in relation to the psychopathology of the patient group and providing extra support for new starters who may be particularly vulnerable to being pulled out of their professional role by patients. Importantly, forensic mental health nurses work within teams and it is crucial that their work remains firmly located within a team approach to patient care and treatment. Teamwork must be both intra- and interdisciplinary with group reflective practice aiming to understand the impact of the patients' psychopathology on the team as well as the individual practitioner. These clinical processes and practices would have as their overall aim the support of nurses working within forensic settings to adhere to the NMC Code (Nursing and Midwifery Council 2008) and maintain the values of the nursing profession while working with a patient group whose emotional impact has the potential to unbalance those with whom interpersonal relating occurs.

RECOVERY

The Department of Health review of mental health nursing concluded with the publication of a strategy for nursing within the United Kingdom which promoted the recovery approach (Department of Health 2006) as a way for nurses to best meet the needs of people with mental health problems. The question to be asked is how applicable to a forensic content are the recovery principles of promoting social inclusion, valuing patients' own treatment aims, embracing hope and optimism and working in partnership? These principles may appear to present particular challenges for nurses working with forensic patients who may be detained indefinitely or who present with particularly complex needs which are hard to treat and whose aims may be to be discharged from care despite being assessed as still presenting a high risk of re-offending. However, it could be argued that the principles of recovery are applicable to this population because recovery is defined as an internal process involving a personal and hopeful journey that the patient makes at their own pace, towards reclaiming a meaningful life from the despair of mental ill health. Instead of withdrawal, dependency and hopelessness which often accompany mental ill health, the process of recovery involves active coping and engagement within the world (Ridgeway 2001). Recovery does not necessarily mean a complete return to wellness although this may happen. However, the mental health practitioner can, by their behaviour, either assist or obstruct the patient in their recovery (Onken *et al.* 2002). Social inclusion aims to enable people with mental health problems to contribute to their communities (Deegan 1988), however community may be defined for each individual. Bates *et al.* (2006) have developed a way to classify mental health day services in terms of the extent to which they are socially inclusive. The classification system is based on the three colours of UK traffic lights. RED = places for disabled people which are used only by patients and staff, AMBER = places that are used by members of the public but groups held there are for patients only, GREEN = shoulder to shoulder with the general public.

The question of how applicable recovery principles are to people detained in forensic services who may have offended seriously as well as having mental health problems might hinge on the extent to which it is realistic to expect that they will ever live independently in the community or 'shoulder to shoulder with the general public'. Certainly, there are a minority of patients in the high security psychiatric hospitals who cannot ever expect to live a life beyond the confines of those institutions because of the risk they present to the public. However, there is no reason why forensic patients should be excluded from recovery-oriented care and treatment. Even people who cannot expect to live within a community setting can be supported and empowered to achieve a meaningful life within a secure setting. The relevance of incorporating a psychodynamic perspective into the work of forensic mental health nurses would aim to maintain the integrity of therapeutic work by enabling nurses to better manage their relationships with patients and maintain a safe, structured and boundaried environment within which the clinical task can be best achieved. In other words, by recognizing the unconscious motivations underlying difficult challenging behaviours, maintaining the capacity to think rather than act out on patients' projections, containing potentially destructive dynamics within the group and the team, being aware of one's own reasons for entering into the field of forensic mental health nursing, a recovery oriented approach is more probable than when any or all of those criteria are absent from a clinical service.

CONCLUSION

The intensely painful emotional circumstances that have often characterized the early developmental experiences of forensic patients can be hard to hear about. Neglect, abandonment and maltreatment of the vulnerable by those tasked with providing love, care, security and protection is always difficult to comprehend whether we are witnessing these horrific relational contexts from the perspective of victim or perpetrator. Yet if we work in the forensic field, such perverse relational material remains live and is played out on a day-to-day basis. In these circumstances, it is the clinician's task to process this difficult aspect of the human condition in order to provide the care, support and treatment forensic patients require if they are to safely recover their lives and at the very least achieve stability and a meaningful experience in a secure setting if discharge is legally prohibited. For nurses, this means having a model of care that enables them to work therapeutically with the disturbing feelings that often occur as a result of close interpersonal relating with the patients in their care. A psychodynamic perspective integrated into their work can offer a helpful way of making sense of the emotional context of their work in a way that may not otherwise be available. This is because much of the emotional disturbance nurses may experience during the course of their work is unconsciously communicated by patients who have no other way of letting their carers know what they are struggling with emotionally. An understanding of projection helps nurses to gain an insight into their patients' needs. The clinical application of psychological containment, including the implementation and maintenance of boundaries in the nursing role, enhances the caring function while reducing the type of acting out that can undermine the therapeutic milieu. For patients with especially complex needs, this paradigm may offer hope and a way to move forward when many other therapeutic modalities alone have not been sufficient to support their needs. For nurses, the application of psychological containment may offer an opportunity for enhanced creativity in their work and a chance to make a difference to populations who are considered especially challenging because of the complexity of their care-seeking behaviours.

In order for nurses to contain patients' projections and use their emotional experiences to inform effective plans of care, they need containing structures to be embedded within the clinical environments as part of the overall treatment provision for patients. Clinical supervision and reflective practice are spaces where thinking about clinical experience can take place. By processing emotional reactions to patients in these spaces, nurses can identify the dynamics of therapeutic relating and use the knowledge gained from this to inform their interventions with patients. In the absence of this type of supportive, containing structure for nurses, the risk is that they will avoid interpersonal contact with patients, becoming emotionally unavailable. Alternatively, nurses may become overwhelmed by their interpersonal experiences in the workplace. Because the emotional content of patients' projections within forensic services usually involves affect associated with abusive experiences, it is particularly difficult to process especially if professionals have their own unresolved vulnerabilities in this regard.

Nursing occurs within a team context. However, the extent to which nurses remain in interpersonal contact with patients makes their role unique.

In order for the nursing role to function effectively, multidisciplinary teamworking needs to support the nursing role by, for example, participating in mixed professional supervision groups and attending ward community meetings. These practices would aim to share the emotional burden and close down the likelihood of destructive projections within the team context which risk replicating the dysfunctional family dynamics that patients experienced during their early development. Multidisciplinary reflective spaces also have the potential to identify and work with splitting which often occurs between different disciplines working in the forensic field. Importantly, general management within these services can support the work of nurses by recognizing their work as emotionally challenging and as a result validating and prioritizing supportive structures required to enable effective clinical work to take place within the emotionally complex world of forensic mental health services.

REFERENCES

Aiyegbusi, A. (2004) '"Nursing under Fire": The Challenge for Forensic Mental Health Nurses Working with Women in Secure Care.' In Jeffcote, N. and Watson, T. (eds) *Working Therapeutically with Women in Secure Mental Health Settings.* London: Jessica Kingsley Publishers.

Bates, P., Gee, H., Klingel, U. and Lippmann, W. (2006) 'Moving to inclusion.' *Mental Health Today,* April, 16–18.

Brown, R. and Stobart, K. (2008) *Understanding Boundaries and Containment in Clinical Practice.* London: Karnac.

Cox, M. (1996) 'Psychodynamics and the Special Hospital: "Road Blocks And Thought Blocks".' In Cordess, C. and Cox, M. (eds) *Forensic Psychotherapy: Psychodynamics and the Offender Patient.* 2 vols. London: Jessica Kingsley Publishers.

Davies, R. (1996) 'The Interdisciplinary Network and the Internal World of the Offender.' In Cordess, C. and Cox, M. (eds) *Forensic Psychotherapy: Crime, Psychodynamics and the Offender Patient.* 2 vols. London: Jessica Kingsley Publishers.

Deegan, P.E. (1988) 'Recovery: The lived experience of rehabilitation.' *Psychosocial Rehabilitation Journal 11,* 11–19.

Department of Health (2006) *From Values to Action: The Chief Nursing Officer's Review of Mental Health Nursing.* London: Department of Health Publications.

Freud, S. (1905) *Fragment of an Analysis of a Case of Hysteria ('Dora').* Standard Edition, Vol. 7. London: Hogarth.

Gabbard, G.O. and Lester, E.P. (1995) *Boundaries and Boundary Violations in Psychoanalysis.* Arlington, TX: American Psychiatric Publishing, Inc.

Kirtchuck, G. and Haworth, H. (1996) 'Psychodynamics and the Regional Secure Unit.' In Cordess, C. and Cox, M. (eds) *Forensic Psychotherapy: Crime, Psychodynamics and the Offender Patient.* 2 vols. London: Jessica Kingsley Publishers.

Nursing and Midwifery Council (2008) *The Code: Standards of Conduct, Performance and Ethics for Nurses and Midwives.* London: Nursing and Midwifery Council.

Onken, S.J., Dumont, J.M., Ridgeway, P., Dornan, D.H. and Ralph, R.O. (2002) *Mental Health Recovery: What Helps and What Hinders? A National Research Project for the Development of Recovery Facilitating System Performance Indicators.* Alexandria, VA: National Association of State Mental Health Program Directors and the National Technical Assistance Center for State Mental Health Planning.

Ridgeway, P. (2001) 'ReStorying psychiatric disability: Learning from first person accounts of recovery.' *Psychiatric Rehabilitation Journal 24,* 4, 335–43.

Temple, N. (1996) 'Transference and Counter-transference: General and Forensic Aspects.' In Cordess, C. and Cox, M. (eds) *Forensic Psychotherapy: Crime, Psychodynamics and the Offender Patient.* 2 vols. London: Jessica Kingsley Publishers.

CHAPTER 2

Managing Hate: The Nurse's Counter-Transference

Malcolm Kay

INTRODUCTION

A number of years ago, as a third-year student nurse I started a therapeutic community placement and was given two papers to read. The first was 'The ailment' by Tom Main (1957) and the second was Winnicott's (1947) paper entitled 'Hate in the countertransference'. Both papers have been corner stones in my nursing and psychotherapeutic practice since, especially when working in forensic environments.

What struck me most then as an enthusiastic student was that Winnicott wrote about mothers hating their babies. Not just a forensic few, but most or all. At the time I found it hard to grasp. However, I suggest that many practitioners still do find it a difficult concept. As a supervisor in supervision and in clinical discussions, I have often encountered the nurses' difficulty in understanding why a parent or, more particularly, a mother could hate their child. Often it is easy not to think of such a dynamic and use words such as 'bad', 'evil' or 'psychotic' to explain this phenomenon. To think about hateful feelings in the patient is difficult. For nurses to think about their hateful feelings towards the patient is often impossible or taboo. In this chapter I will suggest that forensic nurses cannot avoid hating their patients at times. I will also suggest that acknowledging and understanding such feelings will make a significant and positive difference to the way nurses are able to deliver care and treatment to patients.

In 'The ailment', Main (1957) introduces the concept of the 'special patient' and describes a small group of patients who elicit and provoke a specific emotional response in medical staff and to a greater extent, the nursing staff of a psychiatric hospital. He suggests that these responses may be connected to internal conflicts in the individual staff that become aroused by the contact with the patients but, more important, suggests that it is also the result of a manifestation of an area of psychopathology in the patients themselves. Main (1957) describes a form of counter-transference reaction that could be of diagnostic importance. I wonder if we have become less forgiving of nurses who become engaged in complex relationships with their patients. In the current climate, unconscious counter-transference reactions are more likely to be seen as 'mistakes' made by the nurse rather than clues to understanding more about the patient.

THE COUNTER-TRANSFERENCE

Issues around maladaptive caring and health professionals who act out pathologically in the nursing role are often high-profile news. Nurses are often reluctant to admit to ordinary difficulties including strong feelings about their patients. This can lead to a suppression of feelings generally and an ignoring of the emotional and psychological needs of both the nurse and the patient.

As in the development of the concept of transference, counter-transference was initially perceived as an obstacle. Any strong or difficult feelings that the therapist had towards their patient were seen as their own unresolved personal difficulties and conflicts.

However, in Paula Heimann's (1950) seminal paper she wrote of how the counter-transference was not only part of the therapy relationship but also part of the patient's personality and the analyst must use their emotional response as a key to the patient's unconscious.

The nurse who can adopt an attitude of free-floating attention, who can observe from a distance or listen with a 'third ear' to discover what may be behind a surface communication, can tune in to the patient and begin to understand what may seem incomprehensible.

It is well documented how the counter-transference usually catches up with us after the fact, such as when the therapist makes a verbal slip or when we find ourselves doing something that we would not normally do. This overlap of patient and helper pathologies can be useful if discussed within a supervisory space. Consequently, an atmosphere of openness is required so counter-transference responses can be of clinical value and not hidden away or masked for fear of being seen as evidence of poor practice.

CLINICAL EXAMPLE 1

I have begun a trial of psychotherapy with a young woman in a long-term secure setting. The patient is prolific in her self-injury and the purpose of therapy is to attempt to understand this. Initially she engages well and after a couple of weeks stops cutting herself, a state of play that continues for three months, until a two-week break over the summer (my annual leave). In the session before the break the patient is uncommunicative and fears she will hurt herself; she complains that nobody likes or understands her on the ward at present. In talking to her about what could help she tells me she could write her feelings down, poetry being something that had helped previously with another therapist. At the end of the session I find myself helpfully supplying my patient with paper and three felt pens from the stationery cupboard. Immediately afterwards I am aware that this is something I have never done before. On her return to the ward my patient swallows one of the pens and inserts part of another into her arm.

In supervision I am able to acknowledge that my wish to be away from work and on holiday was present in the session. I ignored the fact that I was leaving my patient for a time and any potential anger that she may have with me or that her sudden change in mood was in response to my break. Consequently, I lost any opportunity to work with the transference, i.e. how her feelings about the break might link to other earlier abandonments and disappointments. Instead I became helpful and tried to make the situation better.

Most of the time we have to tolerate not knowing what is going on and, in the case of my work with this patient, I allowed myself to be provoked into a premature reaction to reduce my anxiety. At the time this was preferable to staying with painful and difficult feelings. As it happened, I was left with guilty feelings that I had handed my patient a weapon with which to damage herself. My guilt was mixed with rage about being taken advantage of.

WINNICOTT

Winnicott's (1947) acknowledgement of maternal ambivalence, which he defined as the coexistence of hate alongside love, is a vital concept because such ambivalence is inevitable in all live relationships. It includes and is of particular importance to the forensic setting, in the relationship between nurse and patient.

Psychotherapists and psychologists can manage their hate in the structure of a psychotherapy framework, for example seeing the patient once or twice a week and ending each session after 50 minutes. The consultant psychiatrist can increase or change the patient's medication or hand over care of the patient to a junior doctor. The nurse working on the ward, such as the primary nurse and particularly the nursing assistant, often do not have to hand these distancing techniques that are part of a professional framework. The nurse must manage highly complex, intensive relationships day in, day out.

Winnicott (1947) described his analytic setting as providing the medium for growth that had been absent for the patient from infancy. He described a setting that restored the environment so that development could resume. I have always been struck by the analogy Winnicott offers of why children may hate. Of a child from a broken home he says:

> It is notoriously inadequate to take such a child into one's home and love him. What happens is that after a while a child so adopted gains hope, and then he starts to test out the environment he has found, and to seek proof of his guardian's ability to hate objectively. It seems that he can believe in being loved only after being hated. (p.72)

This 'hating appropriately' is a function of a real relationship.

Winnicott, in 'Hate in the countertransference', lists many reasons why a mother is liable to hate her baby. These include 'he is ruthless', treating her like scum, an unpaid servant, a slave. 'He is suspicious, refuses her good food, making her doubt herself, but eats well with his aunt.' 'He shows disillusionment about her' (pp.73–4). According to Winnicott, the task for the mother is to be able to tolerate hating her baby without retaliation.

Winnicott (1947) states 'The most remarkable thing about a mother is her ability to be so hurt by her baby and to hate so much without paying the child out, and her ability to wait for rewards that may or may not come at a later date' (p.74). This mirrors the nurse with the patient who seems to have bypassed the rational therapeutic contract or care plan and who has resisted recovery over a long time span, as well as the patient who despite the best efforts of all concerned, continues headlong into familiar patterns of destructive behaviour. Consequently it is easy to follow that under such stress, nurses or carers may develop maladaptive strategies with their patients. Broadly speaking such strategies fall into two camps:

1. Over-involvement with the patient's distress.
2. Dismissal or rejection of the patient's distress.

Such strategies are often shared out between various members of the patient's care team. Consequently, splits occur both at individual, ward, department and institutional levels, further complicating an understanding of the patient.

CLINICAL EXAMPLE 2

I have been asked to facilitate a nursing supervision group on a secure ward. The nurses felt such a group would function better in an 'off the ward' environment, the reasons being they would be free from distraction and better able to think. I agree in principle but realize arranging ward cover as well as a suitable venue can become logistical nightmares. Miraculously the first meeting becomes viable and is to be a series of regular weekly meetings for the staff on duty on that day.

Prior to the team taking up their seats in the room, there is a degree of excitement. This seems to be to do with the break in routine and being off the ward, as well as the underlying anxiety about this new group.

There had previously been meetings to define the purpose of the group and it is further clarified that we are here to discuss clinical issues from the ward. A senior experienced staff nurse raises the ongoing difficulty of getting a reluctant patient up in the morning. This is a long-term chronic problem: a patient in a urine-swimming bed must be encouraged to get up, bathe and dress or they will lie there for hours. The task is often fraught and can end in conflict.

At one time or another, all the nurses have been assigned this daily task. Despite numerous care plans and help from psychologists and therapists (like myself) they continue to feel it useless and that the patient will always be reluctant to get out of bed and that nothing will change. On asking how the nurses feel about the patient and by suggesting the words 'hate' and 'contamination', I seem to unleash something.

The group becomes almost manic. Jokes are told about piss and shit, which are met with laughter. Fantasy care plans are suggested with varying degrees of sadism. (I find that forensic nurses tend to have a great sense of the macabre and highly developed sense of humour and wit, which is a mature defence against the emotional burden of their work.) As a facilitator I worry about staying aloof and separate but am also aware of being seduced by the humour and the attempts to draw me in. Consequently, the group continues in this vein and I make a half-baked attempt to draw things together at the end by saying something about humour being a way of defending against the difficult task they have with the patient.

In the intervening week, three members of the group ring me independently to apologize, the central issues seeming to be feeling they behaved unprofessionally. They feel I might think they did not take the group seriously and they feel ashamed about the way they spoke about a patient in their care. In the next group I mention the phone calls and we are able to have a healthier discussion. The staff group speak about how attacked and worn down they feel and there is discussion about a staff member who was warned for retaliating verbally to the patient. We are then able to think about how their fears of retaliating and being unprofessional may be inhibiting ordinary contact with the patient and new ways of thinking about the problem.

Michael and Enid Balint (Balint and Balint 1961) wrote that what the doctor feels is actually a part of his patient's illness. Balint-style groups or work discussion groups where nurses present their patients including their counter-transference can be particularly useful in the forensic setting. Exploring emotional reactions (or in other words, counter-transference reactions) within these group settings is a useful format to help nursing teams manage and understand the forensic patient. Such groups operate from the premise that the forensic patient may be more traumatized, cut off or threatened than the nurse, who will have the greater capacity to tolerate difficult feelings. Consequently the nurses will be less restricted than the patients. By exploring the nurses' emotional reaction to clinical material within a supportive, psychoanalytically oriented supervision space, the nurse can then begin to feel and acknowledge what the patient cannot tolerate in him- or herself. In essence counter-transference feelings can be a mirror of what the patient is feeling or doing to the nurse, both consciously and unconsciously.

I have found it common for forensic nurses not to want to know about the patient's offence. If nurses do know about their patients' offences they tend not to know the detail. On the surface this seems a bizarre concept. How can we nurse the patient without being fully informed and aware of the forensic history? In forensic psychotherapy, the patient's offence is seen as a symptom and a major clue to the hidden nature of their difficulties. How can the person be nursed without the nurse not knowing about these difficulties? The offence can be rationalized as 'not my business'. The offence may be seen by the nurses as the business of the psychiatrist, psychologist or probation officer. The patient will often encourage this dynamic, wanting to keep the nurse or primary carer away from the more shameful, difficult parts of him- or herself. On a more basic level, I also see this split as a way for the nurse to manage her hatred. If she were to know the details of her patient's offending, how could she manage to care for and carry out the tasks assigned to her?

The relationships between nurses and patients are multifunctional in nature and prone to idealization and denigration. The nurse must switch from doing practical tasks for the patient to being there for them in an emotional sense. In practical terms, this can mean supervising lunch times one minute and listening to the patient's emotional struggles the next, followed by administering medication and then meeting a patient's relatives. The nurse simply by virtue of their role has a harder task than do other professional colleagues when it comes to managing time boundaries and being punctual. Ward nurses must respond to emergencies, and the community mental health nurse can be stuck in a traffic jam on the way to an appointment in a patient's home. It is also evident on the ward and in the community that the nurse has more than one patient to care for. It is clear then that of all the roles in the helping professions, the nurse's is most akin to that of mother. It is the forensic mental nurse who is given the most complex demanding patient (baby) possible. We are aware then that patients who have psychotic or complex states of mind can be stressful to work with, such patients having the capacity to project their painful states of mind into those who 'nurse' them. A consequence of this is that the nurse is often left feeling hopeless and despairing or hateful and sometimes murderous.

CLINICAL EXAMPLE 3

An experienced community mental health nurse asks for supervision. She has been asked to take on a male patient newly released from prison. The community mental health nurse knows the patient had been jailed for sexual offences against children and that her task is to monitor his mental health. The patient has been suicidal at times during his sentence. No 'in-depth work' is required of him.

The community mental health nurse raises several issues with me. Should she know details about the offences as she prefers not to? How often should she see him? When should she see him? Primarily she worries that she doesn't like the patient – in fact from their one meeting together she told me that 'he makes my skin crawl' and she worries he will pick this up. She wants to know whether you can monitor a person's mental health separate to their offending history.

In our first supervision I talk to her about counter-transference and often how we can only recognize this after the event. This encourages her to tell me that she managed to double-book the patient for his second appointment, which then had to be rearranged. She recognizes this as a form of acting out of her unconscious wish not to see the patient at all. The first appointment had been difficult and in the patient's home, where the nurse felt she had struggled to keep to the agenda of the visit. The patient's girlfriend had been present, but the nurse had insisted all following visits should be in the GP practice. The nurse also begins to talk about her fantasies about what the patient may have done during his offence and felt this was interfering with her focus when with the patient in terms of monitoring his mental health.

Gradually, the nurse becomes more comfortable in expressing negative feelings about the patient during the supervision sessions. She also becomes aware of how much the patient wants to be in control of their meetings and begins to be clear around the boundaries of their meetings, agreeing appointments in advance for set periods of time. However, despite several attempts the nurse is continually thwarted in getting hold of an accurate forensic history from various sources.

Welldon (1997) lists five essential points when considering the personality traits of the forensic patient, stating that they lead us directly into an understanding of both transference and counter-transference phenomena. They are:

1. The need to be in control, which is often immediately apparent.
2. Early experiences of deprivation and subjection to seductiveness makes them vulnerable to anything reminiscent of the original experiences.
3. A desire for revenge expressed in sado-masochism as an unconscious need to inflict harm.
4. Erotization or sexualization of the act.
5. Manic defense against depression. (p.18)

These traits are highly sophisticated, unconscious defensive mechanisms, which help the patient survive in times of extreme conflict, threat and anxiety. The nurse is often the main target of sadistic and intrusive attacks from the forensic patient and there is a frequent switch between idealization and denigration in the relationship. An increasing and unhelpful trend at present seems to be the 'sacking' of the key worker or primary nurse, usually at a point when the patient switches to the position of denigrator. When the patient is handed on to someone else (often with little resistance from the sacked nurse or the care team) real opportunity is lost in exploring what the difficulty is really about, the patient further buries what is usually a deep and chronic depression and a new nurse–patient relationship cycle begins.

CONCLUSION

The forensic patient at times is also a 'hateful patient' and can provoke a range of feelings in the nurse, including, at times, 'hate'. There is an extra burden for the nurse who, without a safe and containing supervision structure, may have to disown or deny the intensity of feeling aroused by working with the patient. The concept of the counter-transference easily extends outside the formal psychotherapy session and is a vital tool in nurse–patient relationships in the forensic setting. Its value is not only to monitor the individual's response to their patient but the responses of the members of care teams and at times of the wider institution as well. Counter-transference reactions also play an important role in diagnosis and in risk assessment and management. When we find ourself hating the patient and wishing them gone or dead we may then begin to grasp the full extent of their own self-hatred and that the patient may also wish to die.

REFERENCES

Balint, M. and Balint, E. (1961) *Psychotherapeutic Techniques in Medicine.* London: Tavistock Publications.

Heimann, P. (1950) 'On countertransference.' *International Journal of Psychoanalysis 31*, 81–4.

Main, T. (1957) 'The ailment.' *British Journal of Medical Psychology 30*, 129–45.

Welldon, E.V. (1997) 'Forensic Psychotherapy: The Practical Approach.' In Welldon, E.V. and Van Velsen, C. (eds) *A Practical Guide to Forensic Psychotherapy.* London: Jessica Kingsley Publishers.

Winnicott, D.W. (1947) 'Hate in the countertransference.' *International Journal of Psychoanalysis 30*, 69–74.

CHAPTER 3

Forensic Systems and Organizational Dynamics

Gillian Tuck

INTRODUCTION

Working in organizations, whatever their size or task, has an emotional impact on those within them and few organizations are more emotionally challenging than those tasked with the care of highly traumatized and traumatizing forensic patients. The toxic environments that characterize many forensic settings add greatly to the emotional stresses inevitable in nursing work. The nurse works for prolonged periods of time in close proximity to people in great psychological pain. Such work can stir up in the nurse both conscious and unconscious anxieties which in turn give rise to defences, some of which inadvertently serve to increase stress rather than reduce it. Nurses, however, are not the only ones who can be affected by the challenging work. Whole teams and organizations can become dysfunctional if no space is made available to consider their psychodynamics. In this chapter I will draw on ideas developed at the Tavistock Centre, a tradition which integrates open systems theory with psychoanalytic concepts. In doing so, I hope to shed light on some of the complex dynamics that become manifest within caring organizations.

All of the case examples and organizations in this chapter are fictitious but aim to represent the systemic and organizational issues that are relevant in forensic mental health services.

OPEN SYSTEMS THEORY

An open system is a system that exists by continually interacting with and adapting to its external environment (von Bertalanffy 1950). The human body provides a good illustration of an open system in that it imports materials such as food, water and oxygen and transforms them through conversion processes into what it requires for self-maintenance, exporting the remains as waste. To achieve the import–conversion–export processes necessary for survival, open systems depend on the appropriate material exchanges taking place between what is inside and what is outside the area concerned. This involves a series of control mechanisms at the system's external boundary, which aim to keep internal conditions more or less stable. This is achieved by continuously providing the system with what it requires. This highlights the importance of the boundary and its control functions, as failure to maintain a balance between the system and its environment could jeopardize the system's survival. Furthermore, within complex systems like the human body, there are a number of open systems operating at any one time. The various tasks performed by each of these sub-systems require management to ensure they operate in a coordinated way that meets the needs of the system as a whole. As such, superior systems must be developed to provide this coordination and ensure the system functions effectively.

These ideas were developed in the field of biology but they are also applicable to groups of people and organizations. Kurt Lewin (1947) first applied them to human systems. His ideas were further extended by Rice and Miller in the 1950s who developed a framework for studying how an organization's various parts relate to one another, how each part relates to the whole and how the whole relates to its external environment (Miller and Rice 1967).

The organization as an open system

Similar to the human body, organizations must attune themselves to the various pressures and demands emanating from their external environment.

An organization cannot shut itself off from its stakeholders. It must continually import and export forms of energy in order to satisfy its mission and continue to exist. For example, a medium secure psychiatric unit imports patients for which the service is allocated funds. The patient is then treated and rehabilitated by conversion processes such as nursing, psychological therapies and medication. When ready, the patient is exported to the community or another more appropriate setting, leaving a vacant bed which is then filled by the next admission. The funds received by the service are used to maintain the system as well as provide the necessary treatment for patients. If, however, the service were to stop responding to external pressures and demands, its survival would be jeopardized. For instance, failure to admit new patients would leave the unit without the necessary income for self-maintenance.

It is likely that the medium secure unit described above would not simply import patients and money. It may have many inputs and outputs and consist of several interrelated departments such as human resources, psychology, security and catering to name but a few. It is also likely that the various tasks performed by these different departments will at times conflict and compete. Consequently, the effective coordination and management of these departments are essential.

The concept of primary task

The way in which an organization's task systems are ordered and resources managed is ultimately determined by the primary task (Miller and Rice 1967). The primary task can be defined as the task which the organization must perform in order to survive (Rice 1963). At first glance this all sounds very simple. However, as Roberts (1994) points out in her chapter entitled 'The organization of work', the concept of primary task is by no means straightforward, as different individuals and departments within the organization may have different definitions of the primary task. Roberts (1994) also describes how defining the primary task accurately and realistically in organizations with multiple tasks, such as those which aim to change and help people, is often a difficult and complicated process.

The complexity afforded by multiple tasks is clearly evident in forensic mental health settings, which are required to be both custodial and rehabilitative, whilst training staff and developing services. It would not be uncommon for more than one task to take priority at any one time, a situation likely to result in conflict and competition. For example, there may be conflict between patient care and the nurses' training and development needs. In addition, the views of the task held by those outside the organization may conflict with the views of those inside. All of these factors make it difficult for the organization to sustain a sense of effective functioning and those within it a sense of being supported and satisfied at work (Menzies Lyth 1979).

Confused systems: Elmstead Hospital

Elmstead Hospital provides care and treatment for adult men suffering from mental illness and/or personality disorder, who require psychiatric treatment in conditions of medium security. Elmstead's description of its primary task is 'to provide a flexible and responsive service that is committed to multidisciplinary working and needs led care for patients'. The hospital has five wards each housing 12 patients, which include one intensive care ward, two acute wards and two rehabilitation wards. Nurses on Albery, the intensive care ward, had for some time been finding their work unbearable. They would complain of feeling devalued, isolated, frustrated and tired, which was reflected in the high sickness levels amongst nurses working on the ward. One recurring theme was the nurses' view of Albery as a dumping ground for the difficult patients other wards did not want to treat.

During ward meetings nursing staff would regularly raise concerns about poor communication and a lack of consistency in the multidisciplinary team approach to patient care. One example they gave involved the ward doctor who they felt regularly overturned the nurse's decisions, undermining their authority with patients. When asked to define their primary task the nurses gave varied responses; a few half jokingly replied 'surviving till the end of the shift'. The rest were fairly evenly split in their views with half saying their role was to provide care and treatment for the more disturbed patients in the hospital until they were well enough to move to another ward. The other half felt their main role was to keep the ward safe and secure, by closely following hospital policies to minimize the risk of patients harming themselves or others. In addition, all nurses expressed frustration that there were no formalized criteria for the admission or discharge of patients to and from Albery ward. The ward manger described a sense of being pulled in every direction, finding himself absorbed in various incidents on the ward. As a result he was unable to complete the tasks he planned to do each day and felt he was no longer able to see the 'bigger picture'.

Discussion

The hospital's use of broad aims rather than an explicit task seems to reflect some of the difficulties inherent in defining the primary task where tasks are multiple and complex (Menzies Lyth 1979; Roberts 1994). Such a vague definition leaves staff with little guidance about what they are required to do and no benchmark against which progress can be monitored (Roberts 1994). It is unsurprising then, that clarity in relation to the primary task was also lacking at ward level. The ward had no available task definition and no specific criteria for patient admissions or discharges. In addition, the nurses had no clear sense of their primary task. As parts of the wider system the nurses were cut off; they did not know how their work related to the task of the ward or to the task of the organization as a whole. This situation, I would suggest, contributed to the communication problems, inconsistency and low morale evident on the ward. Furthermore, the ward manager had lost his position on the boundary, which meant he was no longer able to manage the ward effectively and provide the internal stability it desperately required.

ORGANIZATIONAL DEFENCES

As the example above illustrates, defining the primary task of the organization and its various sub-systems both accurately and realistically is essential for effective functioning. It is equally important for managers to maintain their position on the boundary of the organization or sub-system where they can respond to external demands whilst maintaining internal stability. To achieve this, an 'eye' must be kept on the task at all times and progress monitored in relation to it.

Staying 'on task' is especially difficult within forensic settings, where the very nature of the work is not only draining and disturbing for staff but also continuously changing as well. The emotional labour and instability inherent to these settings often leads to anti-task behaviour as a defence against anxiety evoked by facing the nature of the primary task. These defences initially adopted by individuals can develop into group and organizational defences over time. These defences are sometimes referred to as socially structured defence systems.

The idea of socially structured defence systems was developed by Jaques in the 1950s. He argued that individual members use the organization to fortify internal defenses against anxiety, which through unconscious cooperation leads to the formation of socially structured defence mechanisms. These social defence mechanisms help to determine the organization's structure, culture and mode of functioning (Jaques 1953). Central to this theory is the externalization of individuals' psychic defences. Although individuals feel the anxiety and employ the defences, it is the collusive interaction and agreement between them that, over time, forms the social defence system (Menzies 1960). These unconscious defence mechanisms are manifest in the form of shared attitudes and ways of working with which all members of the organization must comply.

Organizational defences – a hospital study

Menzies (1960) in her study of a nursing service at a London teaching hospital identified a number of defensive strategies that were employed by the nurses to avoid anxieties, particularly those evoked by the primary task. For instance, by splitting up their contact with patients, nurses were able to avoid the pain of having to think about patients as whole people. This was achieved through the use of a task-list system which meant rather than having to work and make emotional contact with a whole person nurses only had to perform a few tasks for any single patient. This task-list system was supported by a number of other strategies which also disrupted the nurse–patient relationship. Examples of such strategies include the categorization of patients to avoid thinking about individuals, the nurses' uniform which served as a barrier and the way patients were described, not by name, but by bed number and illness.

Another example of the nursing service's social defence system in Menzies' (1960) study was the way in which it was organized to reduce anxieties around individual responsibility. The nurses all experienced painful conflict between the responsibility of their role and their wishes to avoid this sometimes unbearable burden by behaving irresponsibly. This conflict was avoided by a collusive system of splitting, projection and denial, which externalized different aspects of the conflict into different groups within the organization. The nurses' irresponsible impulses were split off and projected into their juniors, who were then treated with the severity which that part of the self was felt to deserve. Similarly, the stern and harsh parts of the self were projected into their seniors, who as a result were expected to be harsh disciplinarians. The roles assigned through these projective processes did not remain at a psychic level; the nurses actually acted on them, giving them substance in objective reality. This collusive externalization of internal conflicts illustrates how the socially constructed defence mechanisms employed in the nursing service became part of the hospital structure, culture and mode of functioning.

Defensive structures: Aldwych Lodge

A group of senior nurses at Aldwych Lodge, a low security hospital providing care and treatment for adult women suffering from personality disorder, embarked on a programme of change aimed at enhancing nurses' clinical input into multidisciplinary team meetings, which was felt to be inconsistent and at times very poor. For example, nursing reports tended to provide a commentary of events rather than a detailed summary of patient progress in relation to planned care. Furthermore, the author of the report was not always the patient's primary nurse. Frequent staff shortages and the busy routine meant reports were regularly written at night by nurses who had limited contact with the patient about whom they were reporting. In addition, other disciplines, particularly doctors, complained that nurses were insufficiently aware of important issues regarding their primary patients and frequently presented inaccurate clinical information.

To enhance clinical nursing input into multidisciplinary meetings a number of 'best practice' standards were developed. For example, it was agreed that all primary nurses should provide and where possible present a brief written report on their allocated patient's progress for the weekly ward rounds. This should summarize the patient's progress in relation to their care plans and should include the perspective of both nurse and patient. In addition, the best practice standards recommended primary nurses provide a substantial written report for their patient's six-monthly review meeting called the care programme approach (Department of Health 1990). This report was expected to include a more detailed account of their allocated patient's progress, with clear recommendations for future care. It was agreed that the primary nurse must attend the six-monthly review meeting. To support nurses with these tasks, report templates and checklists were devised.

After the nurses were asked to implement the best practice standards, a pattern of avoidance seemed to emerge. They began absenting themselves from the multidisciplinary meetings by swapping shifts, going sick or booking annual leave. Those who did attend appeared to fall back on old habits, and very few used the templates or guidance provided.

DISCUSSION

This resistance to change may be better understood in terms of socially structured defence mechanisms (Jaques 1953). Menzies (1960) stresses that change in an organization's mode of functioning automatically means changes in the structure of social defences. With this in mind, it would seem that the changes the senior nurses tried to implement challenged the primary nurses' social defences and in doing so created a great deal of anxiety. In order to avoid this intense anxiety the changes were resisted (Menzies 1960).

In a similar way to Menzies' findings in her study, the forensic mental health nurses' task stirs up a great deal of anxiety, the core of which lies in the nurse–patient relationship. The closer and more intense this relationship, the more extreme the anxiety felt by the nurse (Menzies 1960). The 'best practice' standards required nurses to change a number of known ways of working. For example, in order to provide a thorough report on patients' care and future needs, nurses were required to work more closely and collaboratively with patients. This change threatened the nurses' social defence, in which all the madness and dangerousness is kept in the patients and the sanity in the staff (Main 1975). This defence system is driven by a fear of being contaminated with madness and aggression (Hinshelwood 1987).

The proposed changes also expected nurses to be more professionally accountable by taking responsibility for assessing patient progress and making recommendations for future care. This challenged the nurses' defensive strategy of purposeful disempowerment, used to create a situation where very little is expected of them: a defence that served to reduce the unbearable burden of responsibility evoked by the primary task, as well as helping nurses to pass on that responsibility to other disciplines (Menzies 1960). This defensive strategy is particularly interesting because it seemed to stem from a collusive system of denial, splitting and projection which involved other disciplines' not just nursing. The numerous complaints about nurses' performance may suggest that the nursing service was being used to contain other disciplines' negative projections about their own clinical competence. The burden of responsibility associated with the task also evokes anxiety in other professionals. For example, some doctors fear patients under their care will commit suicide, which arouses intense anxieties about death, one's capacity to damage others and doubts about one's abilities to repair (Menzies 1960). The painful feelings and anxieties evoked by the fear of annihilation are then defended against through processes of denial, splitting and projection (Klein 1946). Perhaps the doctors project their insecurities and persecutory feelings into the nurses in a desperate attempt to gain control of the source of danger. The nurses then act objectively on these through protective identification (Klein 1946). Acting out may manifest in a lack of confidence, poor performance and avoidance. These behaviours are then attacked by the doctors, in the form of complaints, denigrating the nurses. As such, both the nurses' and doctors' defences help sustain each another. This type of intense conflict between different disciplines is a common social defence mechanism within organizations, where negative emotions are split off and projected into others. Each group believes it represents something good and that other groups represent something bad or are inferior in some way (Halton 1994).

CONCLUSION

The application of open systems theory to groups and organizations highlights the role of management, in particular its function at the boundary of the system, where work must be done to ensure the appropriate material exchanges take place between what is inside and what is outside the system. This process requires a clearly defined primary task and constant monitoring of that task in relation to both the system and its external environment. However, for an organization to function effectively a clearly defined primary task and effective management alone are not enough. This is especially true in organizations, such as forensic settings, where the use of socially structured defence mechanisms is often pervasive.

When trying to make sense of the complex dynamics in organizations, it is also necessary to understand how the very nature of the organization's task can stir up anxiety in its members. These individual members then use the organization to reinforce their defence mechanisms against anxiety, which by collusion leads to the development of a social defence system.

This system helps to determine the organization's structure, culture and mode of functioning (Jaques 1953). Any change in an organization's mode of functioning will mean a change in the structure of social defences, during which anxiety will be more open and intense (Menzies 1960).

REFERENCES

von Bertalanffy, L. (1950) 'The theory of open systems in physics and biology.' *Science 111*, 23–9.

Department of Health (1990) *Caring for People: The Care Programme Approach for People with a Mental Illness Referred to Specialist Psychiatric Services* (HC (90)23). London: Department of Health.

Halton, W. (1994) 'Some Unconscious Aspects of Organizational Life: Contributions from Psychoanalysis.' In Obholzer, A. and Roberts, V.Z. (eds) *The Unconscious at Work.* London: Routledge.

Hinshelwood, R. (1987) 'The psychotherapist's role in a large psychiatric institution.' *Psychoanalytic Psychotherapy 2*, 3, 207–15.

Jaques, E. (1953) 'On the dynamics of social structure: A contribution to the Psychoanalytical study of social phenomena deriving from the views of Melanie Klein.' *Human Relations 6*, 3–24.

Klein, M. (1946) 'Notes on Some Schizoid Mechanisms.' In M. Klein, *Envy and Gratitude and Other Works, 1946–1963.* London: Hogarth Press and Institute of Psycho-Analysis, 1975.

Lewin, K. (1947) 'Frontiers in group dynamics, Parts I and II.' *Human Relations 1*, 5–41; *2*, 143–53.

Main, T.F. (1975) 'Some Psychodynamics of Large Groups.' In Kegger, G. (ed.) *The Large Group.* London: Constable.

Menzies, I.E.P. (1960) 'A case-study in the functioning of social systems as a defence against anxiety: A report on a study of the nursing service of a general hospital.' *Human Relations 13*, 95–121.

Menzies Lyth, I. (1979) 'Staff Support Systems: Task and Anti-task in Adolescent Institutions.' In I. Menzies Lyth *Containing Anxiety in Institutions.* London: Free Association Books, 1988.

Miller, E.J. and Rice, A.K. (1967) 'Selections from: Systems of Organization.' In Colman, D.C. and Bexton, W.H. (eds) *Group Relations Reader 1.* A.K. Rice Institute Series, 1975. London: Tavistock Publications.

Rice, A.K. (1963) *The Enterprise and its Environment.* London: Tavistock Publications.

Roberts, V.Z. (1994) 'The Organization of Work: Contributions from Open Systems Theory.' In Obholzer, A and Roberts, V.Z. (eds) *The Unconscious at Work.* London: Routledge.

CHAPTER 4

The Best Defence: Institutional Defences Against Anxiety in Forensic Services

Amanda Lowdell and Gwen Adshead

INTRODUCTION

Anna Freud is credited with first describing how people defend themselves from overwhelming anxiety by employing beliefs, values and attitudes that unconsciously relieve anxiety. There are a variety of these individual defences, and they have both conscious and unconscious elements to them (Freud 1963; Vaillant 1995). In the last half century, there has been increasing interest in how *groups* of people deal with anxiety, and whether groups too use defences. Within larger groups, such as organizations, aspects of the organization's work will give rise to feelings of anxiety and conflicts that will need to be dealt with and managed by psychological defences. People's individual defences join together to form collective group defences that in turn can influence the functioning of any individual in the organization; these are known as social defence systems.

Although these social defences are necessary to manage anxiety, there are two problems attached to them: first, the defences can have a negative impact on an individual's capacity to perform their task, and, second, the defence may not contain the anxiety, especially if it is chronic or extreme. In this chapter, we review what is known about social defence systems in health care, and see how it applies to forensic services.

SOCIAL DEFENCE SYSTEMS IN GENERAL NURSING CARE

In 1959, Isabel Menzies commenced a ground-breaking study which has influenced health care staffing and training ever since (Menzies 1960). A psychoanalyst working at the Tavistock Institute of Human Relations, she was asked to review the allocation of student nurses and overall staffing needs of a large teaching hospital with 700 beds. The hospital had a nurse training school and the nurses were required to work across all sites under the leadership of a matron based at the main hospital site. The workforce consisted of approximately 150 trained nursing staff and 500 students.

The senior staff had encountered great difficulty in balancing the training needs of the students with the overall staffing needs of the organization. Many students were not receiving adequate time in a specific clinical area, and some were due to qualify without having all the required experience. Senior staff felt there was a serious breakdown in their system of training allocation and asked for help in reviewing their methods. Menzies approached her study from a 'socio-therapeutic' perspective, whereby the aim would be to enable desired social change.

Menzies utilized a psychoanalytic approach by viewing the difficulties of student nurse allocation as the 'presenting problem'. She interviewed many staff both structurally and informally, and carried out observational studies in some areas. She discovered that the 'actual problem' of staff allocation arose because one third of nurses were not completing their training due to high levels of anxiety and distress; others frequently took time off due to minor illnesses so that the absence/sickness rate was high.

Menzies felt that the nature of the anxiety needed to be understood. Nurses were in contact with pain and suffering on a daily basis, and were required to perform intimate and distasteful tasks which can arouse feelings such as disgust, fear and hatred; they also might arouse feelings of excitement. She suggested that nurses might envy the care their patients received, or hate the patients for failing to get better; and these negative feelings were in conflict with the positive tender values usually associated with nursing. Menzies stated, 'The objective situation [of love and hate] confronting the nurse bears a striking resemblance to the phantasy situations that exist in every individual in the deepest and most primitive levels of the mind' (p.98).

Menzies suggested that collectively the nursing staff developed social defences to enable them to cope with the intolerable feelings aroused by working in difficult and stressful environments. She argued that these were unconscious defences; staff themselves would not be aware of them, so would seek to argue that they were not anxious. They would not recognize necessarily how certain behaviours were a defence against feeling anxiety. One example was decision-making processes, which were always experienced as life-and-death decisions. The anxiety this caused was defended against by nurses performing a variety of ritualistic tasks, such as checking and re-checking every action or decision. Student nurses were not trusted with such decisions, and discouraged from using any form of initiative or thinking; as juniors, they were the group most affected by these task rituals, but were quickly discouraged from becoming more senior.

Another type of social defence was the increasing separation of the nurses from direct contact with patients. The nursing service attempted to protect the nurses from anxiety by allocating them numerous tasks (sometimes as many as 30 in one shift) for numerous patients. This prevented nurses from coming into too much contact with any one patient and their illness (hence protecting them from anxiety), but undermined their role as carers involved in a personal relationship with the patients.

Another example was the denial of the patient as a person by labelling them in terms of their illness or the bed number: patients were not talked about by name, but might be referred to as 'the Liver in bed 6'. It was presented as essential that nurses treated and viewed their patients in the same way, in that it must not matter what illness or patient they were treating. Patient individuality was reduced, and therefore distress about them as people, and distress at their suffering, was reduced. A related aspect was the emphasis on professional detachment: 'good' nurses did not have particular feelings about any one patient, but treated all patients the same.

Equally, nurses were discouraged from being individuals: the use of nurse uniforms served a purpose in that they could be viewed as 'a kind of agglomeration of nursing skills, without individuality; each is thus perfectly interchangeable with another of the same skill level' (p.102). This enabled 'blanket' decisions to be made and avoided any individuality.

Menzies stated that it seemed to be assumed that any caring professional had to learn to detach and control their feelings, and to avoid 'disturbing identifications'. By reducing any individual distinctiveness, attachments would not form between nurses and patients. Another feature of a 'good nurse' was that they were willing to move from ward to ward with no notice, leaving distressed patients behind without a thought. The implicit rationale seemed to be that a student nurse would learn to be psychologically detached if they actually experienced detachment in the form of the sudden ward moves.

The pain and distress this caused the students was implicitly denied by the hospital system, and explicitly criticized as being 'unprofessional'. Nurses would take a brusque and typical 'stiff upper-lip approach' to upsetting feelings, so that students who were exposed to much emotional strain found senior staff to be unsupportive. However, when senior staff members were interviewed by Menzies, they showed understanding towards the students, but seemed unable to handle emotional stress in any way other than by adopting 'repressive techniques'. Traditional nursing roles supported the use of discipline, repression and reprimand from senior to junior staff, and not a kind, sympathetic approach.

Nurses were found to minimize their anxiety by the use of immature defences such as denial, splitting and projection. These immature defences are commonly used by everyone at times of stress, but in the work situation, staff projected unwanted feelings that they could not bear to feel into other members of the nursing team.

For example, teams became split into those nurses who were 'responsible', and those who were seen as 'irresponsible'. The 'responsible' nurses complained that the 'irresponsible' ones needed to be constantly supervised and disciplined, which led to more and more ritualistic checking behaviour, and prevented the 'irresponsible' staff from actually learning to do their jobs in a responsible way. Projection was not confined to fellow staff; anger and frustration of the work was also projected into patients, who were seen as endlessly demanding and troublesome.

Menzies concluded that these social defences operated to help the individual to avoid the experience of anxiety, guilt and uncertainty, but in fact did not relieve anxiety. Staff still felt anxious and distressed, but the social defences meant that they were not allowed to know their feelings or express them. No attempt was made to enable the individual nurses to confront and face their anxieties and distress, and they were therefore unable to develop a capacity to bear these anxieties more effectively. Without a capacity to manage their distress, it was inevitable that staff would drop out of training and leave, leading to the staffing problems that were the 'presenting problem'.

SOCIAL DEFENCE SYSTEMS IN MENTAL HEALTH CARE

Menzies' study was important for a number of reasons. First, she brought psychodynamic thinking into the workplace, in ways which were practically relevant for running caring organizations. Second, she suggested that group/social defences might mirror individual defences, but be intensified by the group process and organizational structures. Third, she was the first to report that professional carers might actually have negative feelings towards those they care for; that caring was not the highly idealized activity it seemed to be.

There were subsequent studies of different environments, recognizing that different contexts might raise different anxieties, and there developed a whole school for the study of organizational change (Miller 1993). Miller and Gwynne found further evidence of social defence systems operating to deal with anxiety during their study of physically disabled and young chronically ill people in residential settings (Miller and Gwynne 1972). They found two distinct approaches of care towards the residents. In some homes there was a liberal approach where residents were regarded as having the capacity to overcome their difficulties and were put under enormous pressure to develop their skills. They called this the 'horticultural model'. This liberal defence denies the true extent of the disability and both staff and residents are encouraged to remain hopeful of physical cures and rehabilitation, even if, in reality, this is unlikely to be achieved. In other settings, Miller and Gwynne found a more paternalistic approach, where residents were regarded as very damaged and in need of complete care. This was referred to as the 'warehouse model'. This humanitarian defence attempts to prolong life by providing good nursing and medical care, but reducing patient autonomy. In this model, the resident is required to accept the staff's diagnosis and treatment offered and to be seen as a 'good patient': 'doctor knows best'.

Both the 'horticultural' and 'warehousing' approaches are considered as social defence mechanisms to protect against the unbearable anxiety and frustration of caring for a group of people who would never recover health, and would always remain to some extent dependent on others. Since independence and autonomy are associated with maturity and health (at least in Western cultures), long-term dependence and reliance on others are associated with child-like states and hopeless impairment. The hopelessness gives rise to fantasies of death: 'The task that society assigns – behaviourally though never verbally – to these institutions is to cater for the socially dead during the interval between social death and physical death' (Miller and Gwynne 1972, p.80).

We have discussed the Miller and Gwynne study at length because of its obvious similarities with long-stay residential psychiatric care. Elizabeth Bott (Bott 1976; Hinshelwood 2001) first applied Menzies' thinking to a psychiatric setting in a study of a long-stay psychiatric hospital, using an anthropological fieldwork method. Bott found a number of conflicting aims of the task of the organization: a need to control the madness that society could not tolerate, a need to provide care for people who required respite from their intolerable difficulties and the need to offer treatment and cure to patients suffering from illness. Although these aims were not compatible, this was either unrecognized or not accepted by the hospital staff.

Bott noted that staff in a long-stay psychiatric hospital had a profound unease about the task they were performing: an awareness of a 'sort of dishonesty' that patients were admitted, allegedly for their own sake, but actually to relieve other people's anxieties. Thus patients and staff were in a no-win situation; the patient might improve, but they were not necessarily accepted as recovered or welcomed on discharge.

Like the staff in general medical hospitals, nursing staff were forced into contact with people who had severe illnesses that caused damage. But in the psychiatric hospital, the illness and damage was mental; patients lost their personal identities. Not only did patients become dependent on the staff and the hospital, it seemed that they might never recover, and staff became frightened of their illnesses and their disabilities. Fear of madness and distaste for mental distress became the norm, and staff would do all they could to avoid contact with the patients as individuals (Main 1977).

In long-stay institutions, staff were unsure whether patients were there for long-term care or for active treatment; nor was it clear who had the power to decide. Conflict and confusion led to apathy and demoralization on the one hand, and either manic activity or minor acts of sadistic acting out on the other. Donati (1989) observed the engagement of nurses with patients on a chronic psychiatric ward as kept to a bare minimum; as 'touch and go'. Keeping the patients at arms' length was a defence against the fear of the impact of madness on the staff, where madness is symbolic for 'death of the mind' (in contrast to actual death and dying as experienced by nurses in general hospitals). She describes the chronic boredom of the patients and the staff, and the occasional manic bursts of activity by staff who visited the ward briefly but then left again, leaving it disappointed and hopeless again.

RESIDENTIAL FORENSIC SETTINGS

By now, it will be clear that nursing staff working in forensic settings are working in organizations remarkably like those described by Bott, and Gwynne and Miller. In other mental health settings, care has moved to the community, and there is emphasis on 'service users' or 'expert by experience', who 'live with mental disorders', and are managed at home as far as possible. However, in forensic psychiatry, there has been an explosion of residential care, with a huge increase in the number of medium secure unit (MSU) beds (McCulloch, Muijen and Harper 2000). Although it was originally anticipated that patients in MSUs would stay no longer than 18 months to two years, it is now clear that the average length of stay in an MSU is closer to five years (Shaw, Davies and Morey 2001). In the high security hospitals (which used to be called 'special': Broadmoor, Rampton and Ashworth), the average length of stay remains at about eight years, although there is a considerable range (Maden *et al.* 1995).

What this means is that forensic staff are now responsible for long-stay residential psychiatric care, with nurses and patients living cheek by jowl for hours of days of weeks of years. Staff in these settings will spend more time with the patients than with their own families; and these units and hospitals can become like enclosed communities of both staff and patients. In one case known to us, both a patient and his primary nurse had entered the hospital at the same time, 23 years previously: they had both 'grown up' together in a high security hospital.

Nursing staff therefore have to manage the demands of long-term care for people with severe mental illnesses. However, they also have to try and make therapeutic relationships with patients who have committed horrifying and disturbing acts of violence against humanity. Normally, people who have done such acts are shunned by others; instead, forensic nurses have to try and care for them, and nurses are faced with this challenge each time they enter the hospital to perform their nursing role. We can imagine, using both Menzies' and Bott's formulations, that staff have to defend themselves not from *unconscious* fear alone, but from *conscious* fear of the patients, who have been identified as highly risky people. The emphasis on security measures means that nursing staff are being encouraged to provide a personally supportive relationship to patients, while at the same time being suspicious of the danger they pose.

Unconsciously, we may imagine that staff fear the madness in the patients, envy their care, and hate the hopelessness that their situation seems to provoke. Defensive manoeuvres include distancing themselves from the patients as much as possible (for instance by withdrawing into the office or kitchen), rubbishing attempts to help the patients (Sarkar 2005), and seeing patients as either 'all good' or 'all bad'. This last issue is clearly an example of splitting, and represents both a manic defence against the reality of what the patients have done, and a cruel identification with the hopelessness of their position.

There are three other problems peculiar to work in forensic residential institutions, which give rise to particular anxieties and defences. First, the vast majority of forensic patients not only have severe treatment resistant mental illnesses, but also suffer from moderate or severe personality disorders. The psychological impact of working with such disordered patients has been well described in the psychiatric literature (Norton 1996), but rarely applied to forensic settings. Patients with personality disorders not only relate socially in immature and fragmented ways; they also elicit care from professional carers in hostile and toxic ways (Adshead 1998; Henderson 1974; Main 1957). In outpatient settings, staff may respond by distancing themselves from the patient (Watts and Morgan 1994); in forensic settings, this may not be possible (Whittle 1997).

Second, the conflict of purpose that Bott described in the old-style asylums is even more intense in forensic institutions. Are the staff there to help the patients feel better or behave better? How can they work towards patient recovery and discharge when it is not at all clear that anyone wants them to be discharged? If they do not provide treatment, patients will be institutionalized and hopeless, and the 'nursing' purpose will be gone; however, if they do not provide long-term care, there will be damaged patients who may end up being abandoned in the community with potentially awful consequences for them and others. This conflict between 'care' and 'custody' is a crucial one for forensic nursing staff, and it leads to a multiplicity of unconscious behaviours that allow avoidance of thinking.

Finally, there is one anxiety that all forensic professionals try and keep as far from consciousness as possible, and that is the fear that we can identify with these violent and cruel patients. This can take the form of excitement over their crimes and pathology, or an excessively punitive stance towards the patients. Robert Simon, a distinguished forensic psychiatrist, wrote a book entitled *Bad Men Do What Good Men Dream* (1996); a contemporary forensic echo of the Kleinian theory described by Menzies.

Both Simon and Mrs Klein would argue that we all have innate feelings of hatred and cruelty that we manage in fantasy; but patients in forensic situations have actually carried those feelings across from the internal to the external world. Those who work with forensic patients may have unresolved feelings of hatred and cruelty that they long to act on, but cannot; they may wish that their capacity for cruelty and violence was cared for in the same way as the patients. This may be especially true for those staff members who have actual histories of childhood victimization. Professionals like ourselves may be drawn to this work because we also unconsciously long to be cruel, or perhaps because we unconsciously seek revenge for past hurts, or because we are unconsciously anxious about our capacity for destructive anger. Whatever the reason, a variety of defensive acting out behaviours by staff may be driven by the anxiety that we psychologically resemble the patients.

MAKING AND MAINTAINING THERAPEUTIC RELATIONSHIPS IN FORENSIC SETTINGS

How is it possible to form therapeutic relationships with individuals who have committed horrific offences, and still have the capacity to act in a violent and dangerous way on and off the ward? Some staff cope by ignoring the offence and the behaviour of such patients, and focus only on their vulnerability. More often, negative feelings towards patients are ignored or unacknowledged, or staff work hard at detaching themselves from such feelings. Since developing psychological detachment from distressing feelings is still seen as a professional nursing skill in general nursing, the potentially harmful consequences of long-term detachment are not considered.

MANAGING ANXIETY

Understanding and managing risk are fundamental to the forensic organization. Robust risk assessments are carried out, updated and referred to constantly. There is an unspoken fear that to miss out any detail could lead to a potential disaster, so the anxiety is huge. The rituals of risk assessment and attention to physical security resemble the rituals Menzies found in her study, but have acquired an extra significance at a time when psychiatric services have been given the impossible task of preventing all possible future harm by a risk-averse society. Doctor (2004) suggests that the belief that risk assessment will avert future violent tragedies has now assumed almost delusional proportions.

However, unlike the nurses observed in Menzies' study, nurses working in the residential forensic setting *do* retain close contact with their patients, as both they and the patients remain in the organization for some considerable length of time. They cannot escape personal relationships with the patients unless they are promoted into management posts, or leave the service. Primary nurses, in particular, are required to develop psychotherapeutic relationships with their allocated patients, which are intended to help the patients talk about their experiences and their feelings. What this means in reality is that nurses have to listen to accounts of both the patients' offences and their personal backgrounds. Since 80 per cent of forensic patients have been childhood victims of extreme abuse (Coid 1992) which has severely traumatized them, the content of what they have to say is usually very disturbing to hear, and staff may not know what to say. Some patients engage in an unconscious symbolic re-enactment of either their abuse or the offence, so that the nurse ends up feeling either like a victim or a perpetrator of abuse. Patients with personality disorders tend to use immature defences as a default way of managing feelings, so that they usually deal with a range of overwhelmingly negative and uncomfortable feelings by projecting them into the nurse who is trying to listen to them.

Patients may relate to nurses as significant parental figures from a patient's past; especially since the nurse is someone who both cares for the patient and controls them, much like earlier attachment figures (Adshead 1998). Nurses can find themselves on the receiving end of rapidly oscillating attitudes from the patients (either needy or hostile) which leave them feeling bewildered and deskilled. For example, a patient with a persecutory and abandoning past care-giver will engage in a hostile way to a nurse who offers support in a kind and concerned way. The nurse experiences a hostile rejection and abandonment, just as the patient experienced in the past, and may be tempted to either abandon the patient, or respond aggressively, much as the past care-giver did. If they do so (and even the best of us may do so), the re-enactment has taken place. It is *essential* that all staff learn to understand this process to prevent further damage to the patient.

REFLECTIVE PRACTICE

One way for staff to learn about projection and re-enactment is to reflect on their work with other professionals. It is psychologically healthy for nurses to give themselves permission and to be encouraged to express their negative feelings about their patients rather than use defences of denial and projection. A helpful forum for nurses to meet to talk about their patients and their own feelings towards them is in a reflective practice (RP) group. Reflective practice is now seen as essential for all those staff working with patients with personality disorders, especially in complex needs or forensic services (NIMHE 2003)

We describe here some material from an RP group for forensic nursing staff. This group meets on a two-weekly basis on a ward within a secure forensic service. The aim of the group was agreed with the nursing staff, and it was decided that the group would act as a space where nurses could be enabled to understand their own reactions to their patients. Staff were particularly interested in why patients seemed to respond and behave so differently to certain members of staff, and it was felt that this would be helpful to discuss. The group membership is diverse in that qualified and unqualified staff, student nurses and the clinical ward manager all attend. It is an evolving group where new members of staff join and others leave.

In the beginning, it was difficult for staff to talk about the feelings that they *actually* had, as opposed to the feelings that they thought they *should* have. For example, one member said that it was her job to care for her patients, regardless of their diagnosis, behaviour or offending history, and that she felt the same way about all her patients. To her, they were all recovering from a mental illness and needed care and understanding; she wished only to understand more about her patients' psychological processes and felt that her own feelings were unimportant.

As the group progressed, the members gradually talked about different feelings towards their patients. One nurse talked about John, who had recently required restraining at regular intervals throughout several shifts to prevent him from injuring himself in a particularly disturbing way. His attacks on himself seemed relentless. Other staff joined in the discussion, some expressing their frustration and anger and others saying how awful it was to be waiting for the next act of self-harm. Some staff reflected on how terrible it must be for him, whereas others felt he was 'conning' staff and was not suffering emotional distress that much. There was anger amongst some staff in that he pushed them away, making it impossible to have a therapeutic relationship with him because he would not allow any contact. They felt useless, rejected and unable to fulfil their nursing role as 'carer'.

There seemed to be an emotional outpouring from the group members and a desperate need to fix things and make everything all right for the patient, and, at an unconscious level, for themselves. It seemed unbearable to be able to tolerate his distress. One member said she would 'never give up on him' and was determined that he would stop his destructive behaviours. Several members said he would be 'better off' somewhere else where specialist staff would be more skilled to deal with him. These feelings of helplessness were passed around all the staff including the clinical team, but the unspoken message seemed to be a desperate plea of 'Please take him away so that we'll be less worried and the ward will become a safe place once again.'

The anxiety within the group was palpable, and the room seemed to contain a mass of expressed diverse emotions. Fear was not verbally expressed but seemed to be very present, both for John and for the staff. They were asked to think about whether their own feelings of fear could be feelings projected from John; whether he could not bear to own his difficult to manage and unbearable feelings, so had unconsciously projected them onto his carers. The group explored the possibility that their role in caring might be in 'holding' the patient's emotional distress, and that this is a difficult task that needs sharing and understanding. If the nurses can consciously bear John's intolerable feelings in their own minds without taking any destructive action, this might enable some form of psychological safety for him. Further, if his difficult and troublesome feelings are held safely and knowingly (i.e. the nurses are consciously aware of this process), then they can start to be talked about openly and his ongoing risk can be better managed.

This patient was often talked about in the group subsequently. The concept of 'splitting' was explored where members were able to think in more depth about these different aspects of John, their feelings and the part they played in his care. During one group session, it was announced, 'there's been a change in John.' A week had passed with no incidents of destructive behaviour and he had begun to communicate with the staff. Some members were wholly optimistic and jubilant; others were more cautious about this change, and the significance of carrying hope for such a damaged and abused patient was explored. The group was asked to think about the possibility that some patients may not be 'cured' and that delivering effective therapeutic nursing care in forensic settings might be sometimes akin to palliative care, i.e. the management and relief of pain and discomfort rather than curing the source of the pain.

John remained on the ward and continued to be successfully and sensitively cared for by the staff. He has been spoken about and reflected on in many group sessions and there is a general sense of clearer awareness and deeper understanding of him and his carers.

CONCLUSION: SOMETHING UNDERSTOOD: THE DEMANDS OF FORENSIC MENTAL HEALTH NURSING

Are nurses working in forensic residential settings simply mental health nurses working in a psychiatric setting where the patients stay longer and have committed an offence? Or is there something different about the environment and the patients and therefore something different is required of the nurses?

We hope that we have made it clear that there is something extra that has to be understood about the role of forensic nurses in long-stay residential settings, such as secure units. The forensic residential setting represents a place of containment and safety, for the patient and for society. Physical security is paramount and the locking of doors and risk management plans are essential to contain the patient and to reduce the anxiety. However, it is also evident that *psychological* security is important, not only to manage the seriously damaged and traumatized offenders residing within, but also to assist the staff in this most demanding task of both caring for and containing potential violence.

We hope to have shown how Menzies' original study has important implications for forensic nursing, especially in relation to thinking about the index offence that brought the patient to the hospital or prison. In Menzies' study, the patient's experience of illness or disease was not thought about as one way of managing anxiety. In forensic settings, both staff and patients try to avoid thinking about the index offence, and the anxiety it brings. The offence must not be forgotten about, but at times it seems to be 'lost' unconsciously, as to think about it might make it unbearable for the staff to 'care' for their patient. This 'forgetting' or disavowal is a mirror of the patients' wish (both consciously and unconsciously) to forget the offence. Hence it is possible for a patient in a forensic setting never to discuss their index offence during their stay.

Menzies' original work needs to be understood and integrated with other theoretical advances over the last 50 years, especially research in the field of traumatic stress reactions, the impact of childhood trauma on neurological development and attachment theory as a theory of care-giving. If we understand that social defence systems act to make organizations feel psychologically secure, and to make individual staff the carriers of intolerable anxiety, then this might assist us to put in place structures and policies that help staff and organizations reduce destructive acting out. This in turn will help care-giving organizations, such as forensic psychiatric services, the chance to become more resilient (Kahn 2005). The extent of the anxiety felt in forensic institutions should not be underestimated, as unconsciously indicated by the message on a sign hung on the canteen in a forensic unit: 'This building is alarmed'.

Acknowledgements and disclaimer: thanks to colleagues at Broadmoor and Ravenswood House Medium Secure Unit for space to discuss these issues in peer supervision meetings. Although the material is clinically accurate, names and details have been changed to protect staff and patient confidentiality.

REFERENCES

Adshead, G. (1998) 'Psychiatric staff as attachment figures.' *British Journal of Psychiatry 172*, 64–9.

Bott, E. (1976) 'Hospital and society.' *British Journal of Medical Psychology 49*, 97–140.

Coid, J. (1992) 'DSM II diagnoses in criminal psychopaths; the way forward.' *Criminal Behaviour and Mental Health 2*, 78–95.

Doctor, R. (2004) 'Psychodynamic lessons in risk assessment and management.' *Advances in Psychiatric Treatment 10*, 267–76.

Donati, F. (1989) 'A psychodynamic observer in a chronic psychiatric ward.' *British Journal of Psychotherapy 5*, 317–29.

Freud, A. (1963) *The Ego and the Mechanisms of Defence.* London: Hogarth.

Henderson, S. (1974) 'Care eliciting behaviour in man.' *Journal of Nervous and Mental Disease 159*, 172–81.

Hinshelwood, R.D. (2001) *Thinking about Institutions: Milieux and Madness.* London: Jessica Kingsley Publishers.

Kahn, W. (2005) *Holding Fast: The Struggle to Create a Resilient Care Giving Organisation.* London: Brunner Routledge.

Maden, T., Curle, C., Meux, C., Burrow, S. and Gunn, J. (1995) *Treatment and Security Needs of Special Hospital Patients.* London: Whurr.

Main, T. (1957) 'The ailment.' *British Journal of Medical Psychology 30*, 129–45.

Main, T. (1977) 'Traditional psychiatric defences against close encounters with patients.' *Canadian Psychiatric Association 22*, 457–66.

McCulloch, A., Muijen, M. and Harper, H. (2000) 'New developments in mental health policy in the UK.' *International Journal of Psychiatry and the Law 23*, 261–76.

Menzies, I. (1960) 'A case study in the functioning of social systems as a defence against anxiety: A report on a study of the nursing service of a general hospital.' *Human Relations 13*, 95–121.

Miller, E. (1993) *From Dependency to Autonomy: Studies in Organisation and Change.* London: Free Association Books.

Miller, E. and Gwynne, G. (1972) *A Life Apart.* London: Tavistock.

NIMHE (National Institute for Mental Health in England) (2003) *The Personality Disorder Capabilities Framework.* Leeds: NIMHE.

Norton, K. (1996) 'Management of difficult personality disorder patients.' *Advances in Psychiatric Treatment 2*, 202–10.

Sarkar, S.P. (2005) 'The other 23 hours: Special problems of psychotherapy in a "Special" hospital.' *Psychoanalytic Psychotherapy 19*, 4–16.

Shaw, J., Davies, J. and Morey, H. (2001) 'An assessment of the security, dependency and treatment needs of all patients in secure services in a UK health region.' *Journal of Forensic Psychiatry and Psychology 12*, 610–37.

Simon, R.I. (1996) *Bad Men Do What Good Men Dream: A Forensic Psychiatrist Looks at the Darker Side of Humanity.* Arlington, TX: American Psychiatric Publishing, Inc.

Vaillant, G. (1995) *The Wisdom of the Ego.* Boston, MA: Harvard University Press.

Watts, D. and Morgan, G. (1994) 'Malignant alienation: Dangers of patients who are hard to like.' *British Journal of Psychiatry 164*, 11–15.

Whittle, M. (1997) 'Malignant alienation.' *Journal of Forensic Psychiatry and Psychology 8*, 5–10.

CHAPTER 5

The Dynamics of Difference

Anne Aiyegbusi

INTRODUCTION

In this chapter, it will be argued that forensic mental health services have a long history of struggling to provide safe therapeutic care, especially to those patients who are members of minority groups. A surprising aspect of services for mentally disordered offenders is that, despite good intentions and often admirable efforts, progress is usually remarkably slow and difficult to achieve. Some of the struggles to meet the needs of minority groups within services have been evident in the maltreatment and deaths of patients, reaching the public domain in the form of inquiry reports such as *Big, Black and Dangerous* (SHSA 1993), the chapter entitled 'Women in Ashworth' within the Blom-Cooper Inquiry into abuse of patients at Ashworth special hospital (Department of Health 1992) and the Rocky Bennett Inquiry (Department of Health 2003). An unfortunate consequence of reports such as these and the tragedies that precede them is that, on the surface, the ubiquitous problem of discrimination of the grounds of difference gets identified with a small number of isolated services, events and individuals.

Changes that emerge from public inquiries, similar investigations and reviews inevitably focus on structural and social domains. The implementation of strategies to address the behaviour of employees is seen as central to the achievement of change. Much needed as such action is, there is a danger that thought remains the same only to become enacted at a later date. The observation of particular themes recurring decade after decade suggests a need to also explore the psychological processes that underpin discrimination within forensic institutions.

Several authors have argued that social explanations for discrimination on the basis of difference offer an incomplete analysis. Clarke (1999), Bird and Clarke (1999), Dalal (2002) and Frosh (2005) suggest that a psychological dimension is also required in order to achieve a more complete understanding of racism, sexism, homophobia and other 'hate' phenomena. They argue that the social expression of prejudice is underpinned by conscious and unconscious psychological processes that are inherent within the human condition. This chapter will describe the psychodynamic processes that are central to understanding human beings' propensity to discriminate against one another, sometimes in hateful, hurtful ways. Why forensic mental health services may be prone to the creation of environments characterized by painful interpersonal relating that usually involve various forms of attacking difference will be explored in this chapter. Nursing processes and practices that aim to work thoughtfully and effectively with the dynamics of difference will also be described in this chapter.

THE PARANOID-SCHIZOID POSITION

Klein (1946) introduced the concept of the paranoid-schizoid position, an early psychological defence against anxiety whereby the self becomes deeply split into good and bad parts. Good parts represent the life instinct and bad parts are associated with the death instinct. Difference as represented by good and bad parts of the self cannot be held together within the mind because of overwhelming anxiety. In the paranoid-schizoid position, good parts of the self are usually retained but bad parts of the self, which are felt to be unacceptable, have to be evacuated and so are unconsciously projected onto a suitable object, invariably another person. The other person who functions as a receptacle for unwanted projections is then experienced as embodying those unpalatable characteristics. This enables the projector to witness their unwanted qualities from a distance, within another who can then be interacted with disdainfully. An example would be of a young man struggling with his sexuality who makes homophobic comments towards a gay acquaintance, insinuating that same-sex relationships are unnatural.

Projective identification

Klein's theory of the paranoid-schizoid position also described the powerful, primitive defence mechanism of projective identification. In projective identification, the person projects 'into' rather than 'onto' another, applying interpersonal pressure until the other experiences the projections as part of themselves. To return to the example of the young man struggling with his sexuality, projective identification could result in his gay acquaintance feeling that his own sexual feelings were abnormal and seeking counselling as a result. Bion (1959) has described two kinds of projective identification. The first involves communicating mental states to other people. The second type of projective identification that Bion (1959) describes can be violent and raw. This involves forcing out unpalatable, unprocessed parts of the self, until they become felt by another person. Typically, the other is forced to contain uncomfortable emotional states which can be as extreme as terror, rage and murderousness. Bird and Clarke (1999) emphasize the affective nature of projective identification and suggest that, as an interpersonal process, it provides a model for aggressive relating. As such, it may serve as a useful model for understanding the interpersonal transaction between victim and offender. For example, Gary is convicted of attempted murder and detained in a high security psychiatric hospital. In therapy he described how, when he looked into the eyes of his victim while holding a knife to her throat, he knew that at last somebody understood what it felt like to be him. The forensic patient in this example had been regularly terrorized as a child and had on numerous occasions felt sure that he would be killed during beatings by his violent stepfather. Overwhelmed by his terror and compelled to re-enact his trauma, the only apparent means available for him to communicate this unprocessed experience was by forcing the affect into another person to feel his terror as their own.

HATRED AND OTHERNESS

As Horwitz (1983) points out, when it is understood that through interpersonal interactions people 'may transfer mental contents from one another and back and forth we appreciate the full complexity of behaviour in a group setting' (p.269). Not only do people project unwanted parts of themselves into others, but the other can feel and act in accordance with those projections, experiencing them as part of themselves and this can happen between individuals, and within groups and societies on the basis of which cultures are defined. With regard to racism, Fanon (1952) describes the experience of being black and imprisoned in a world constructed by white men. In this world, racist phantasies are intense and through the mechanism of projective identification are forced into black people whose lived experience now concurs with the content of those projections. Thus, the black person who has been projected into then experiences themselves as a denigrated being and behaves accordingly. In turn this maintains the racist view held by white people. Thus, a cycle of black failure within a white culture becomes perpetuated.

An important aspect of discrimination and bigotry is that by projecting unpalatable parts of the self into a denigrated other, the phantasy of the self as all good is maintained. Therefore, there is an implicit and often necessarily enduring relationship between the projector and their target. One is needed to maintain the psychic equilibrium of the other which may explain the powerful resistance that tends to accompany efforts to change discriminatory actions on the one hand and thoughts on the other. Change with regard to the latter is rarely even broached especially in relation to addressing the unconscious processes that maintain oppression on the basis of difference. One reason for this might be that projection operates both at the level of the racist, for example, and among those who serve to challenge racism. In the latter group, it may be more comfortable to think of the other as delinquent while the self is maintained as all good and innocent of any potential for bigotry. Increasing self-awareness would lead to an appreciation of the ubiquity of projection and the fact that everybody unconsciously disposes unwanted parts of themselves onto others in one form or another, especially when exposed to high levels of stress, anxiety or fear. A development has occurred in recent years with regard to race though. That is, the allegation of racism now appears to hurt to a degree that it appears to approximate the hurt caused by racist behaviour. Thus, in forensic environments one group of people may be in fear of 'the race card' in the same way that others fear the racist act.

Frosh (2005) has elaborated upon the relationship between projector and target from the perspective of racism and anti-Semitism and suggests that in order for cultures to maintain their civility those parts of the psyche that live within all of us and may be regarded as primitive but alien, have to be projected into another group for 'civilized' cultures to be maintained. Frosh (2005) goes so far as to suggest that the unconscious longings and desires that inhabit all people are subjectively experienced as alien. What is projected into externally alien groups gives a clue about what our unconscious longings and desires consist of. Generally speaking these projections may include phantasies about socially undesirable indulgencies, such as unrestrained hedonism, incompetence, danger, greed, sloth, unbridled sexuality and irresponsibility. Frosh (2005) questions whether this internal, alien part is actually what governs the minds of people rather than the more sophisticated, rational, evolved or conscious part of the human psyche. This formulation could also explain the relationship between forensic patients and nurses in that the patients may provide a convenient container for nurses' unconscious phantasies, enabling nurses to function more comfortably in the social world. Because they are identified as a group who have actually acted out the phantasies other people have, this population may be particularly appealing to the unconscious in terms of serving as repositories for nurses' alien other. For the same reasons, forensic patients as a group who employ primitive defence mechanisms, such as splitting, projection and projective identification, can often be an emotionally difficult population to work with. For the patients, difference has so often served as a target for attack and annihilation as unwanted, internally alien affect is unconsciously deposited in the other. This pattern of interpersonal relating is present within the forensic organization that is uncontained and unable to think about unconscious processes operating within professional groups. In such cases, professionals replicate the style of interpersonal relating that is central to the forensic patients' psychopathology, including attacking and annihilating difference.

One of the factors making caring for forensic patients so complex is that they are victims as well as perpetrators of violence. Therefore, projections are likely to include emotional material associated with victimhood as well as perpetration. The bullying interpersonal transactions that pervade services, often on the part of nurses and other professionals as well as the patient group, can be understood in terms of sado-masochistic functioning. Because nurses work in close proximity to patients, they are often required to process raw and intense sado-masochistic projections (Temple 1996). When nurses are not able to manage this difficult task, they act out on the material, engaging in bullying and discrimination. As such, some nurses adopt the more sadistic role as bully, racist or homophobe for example, while others are on the receiving end of these painful interpersonal interactions.

Case example

Due to chronic nursing shortages, an NHS trust in the United Kingdom made a determined effort to recruit a large number of staff from overseas. The NHS trust was located in a part of the country where the population were mostly white and UK born. The newly recruited overseas nurses were not white. Many of these nurses were allocated to work in the local forensic services where nursing shortages had been of particular concern. Their presence was met with emotionally violent rejection and denigration from the patients. The overt abuse and denigration centred on the nurses' physical appearances; that is, those characteristics that were seen as different from their own. Also, the patients on this unit denigrated the overseas nurses' clinical skills as did many of the local nursing staff. Despite having high levels of training and successful careers elsewhere, this cohort of newly recruited nursing staff became hesitant in their work and were reluctant to engage with the patients. As a result, they were further criticized for not being able to do their jobs and became identified within the organization as a group with inferior skills who needed extra supervision.

Discussion of case example

The above case provides an example of how observable difference, on this occasion racial, provides a convenient repository for group projections based on existing feelings of inferiority and denigration within local nurses and the patients. The disorientation of the overseas nurses, who were required to make a huge adjustment to a new country and culture in addition to fresh working arrangements, provided existing, demoralized nurses with an opportunity to be relieved of the emotional burden of feeling devalued and inferior. The overseas nurses also provided the forensic patients with an easy receptacle to contain their hard to manage feelings such as fear, vulnerability, alienation and incompetence in terms of failing to succeed in life. Through the application of interpersonal pressure, the overseas nurses began to experience the projected feelings as their own and acted on them, making mistakes and hesitating to get involved with patients. The organization joined in the painful scenario and responded concretely by providing extra supervision. The supervision was not intended to enable the nurses to understand what was going on from a psychological perspective but simply to produce change on a practical or social level in terms of improved performance. In turn, this managerial intervention compounded the discrimination. This example demonstrates how difference can so easily serve as a template for sado-masochistic relating, especially within forensic services as patients and professionals unconsciously seek out receptacles to contain their disturbing feelings.

A thoughtful approach to managing the dynamics of difference

An alternative scenario to that described in the above case example might involve a forensic service with commitment to providing a culture of enquiry (Griffiths and Leach 1998) enabling the local nurses, overseas nurses and patients to understand what was going on within their relationships. Community meetings are forums where patients could be challenged about their projections. For example, in a similar unit where patients were racially abusing a new group of nurses the patients were asked in their community meeting whether having to rely on a new group of nurses for care made them feel particularly vulnerable. Thinking about their feelings of vulnerability in a safe space resulted in some of the patients talking about how worried they were about the new nurses reading their case notes before getting to know them. This anxiety was acknowledged by the group as a whole when one patient was able to explain how frightened he was feeling about being looked after by people he did not know. This patient described having a number of experiences in his life when he had been 'handed over to strangers'. Each experience of simultaneous separation/introduction felt like a catastrophe. Nurses and patients were able to think about how it would also be easier for the patients to pull the nurses out of their roles rather than wait to be failed by them. Applying so much pressure onto the nurses was one way for patients to take control of their relationships with care-givers. By corrupting the nature of care provided, the patients would be in familiar territory, therefore assuaging anxiety arising from vulnerability.

The new nurses were able to reassure patients that they would organize a number of introductory one-to-one sessions with their primary patients. This would enable the patients to discuss their histories and current needs. The new nurses agreed to involve the patients in any decisions about care plans and would avoid making any radical changes to existing programmes until both parties agreed that a therapeutic rapport had been established. The nurses also clearly communicated the boundaries between their roles and that of the patients, what their authority was and the limits of what would be tolerated in terms of antisocial expressions of distress.

The overseas nurses were supported in their strategy of care by their colleagues. The new and established nurses were able to work as a team in confronting the patients' feelings and behaviour because they had previously been able to explore their own relationships and associated anxieties safely in regular, externally facilitated staff groups. By acknowledging their anxieties together, the two groups of nurses had established common ground, which enabled them to focus on the primary task of delivering health care to patients. By remaining on task as a team, progress could also be made with regard to improving the reputation of the service within the wider organization. Nurses were able to recognize that engagement in perpetual conflict enabled them to avoid anxieties associated with the primary task (Menzies Lyth 1988). In forensic mental health nursing, such anxieties arise from close emotional engagement with patients' distress and destructiveness.

By exploring the unconscious processes underlying uncomfortable affect on the part of nurses and patients, what was going on within the social environment was clarified and therefore possible to work with creatively rather than destructively. However, such a challenging task could not have been achieved without a psychologically oriented management team (Obholzer 1994) who approached the appointment and integration of a large group of overseas nurses carefully and with sensitivity to the impact their appointments would have on the patients, the nurses themselves and their colleagues. As such, the action involved in the appointments alone was not seen as the complete solution to the staffing problems. The effective solution required thought on the part of management and the ability to understand the importance of addressing unconscious organizational processes associated with patients' psychopathology as well as observable social behaviour in order to achieve change (Obholzer 1994). Additionally, by being afforded an opportunity to process their feelings together, overseas and local nurses were able to think about hostilities within both groups. By both parties acknowledging their fantasies and feelings of hostility towards each other, as well as their uncertainties and vulnerabilities, neither group was inclined to adopt the role of victim or perpetrator.

TWO TRIBES

The suggestion that discrimination in forensic services only occurs between people who are of different races is to miss the point. While race does appear to provide a particularly convenient receptacle for certain types of projections, it is by no means the only form of difference to emerge as central to in-house conflicts. Gender, sexuality, profession or grade will serve just as well. These apparently tribal conflicts are typical in forensic services for a number of reasons. Forensic patients sometimes function exclusively in the paranoid-schizoid position with extreme use of splitting and projection which is hard for nursing staff to process through thought rather than action. The most obvious split involves the victim/perpetrator dynamic. It is very difficult to integrate the fact that most forensic patients are both victim and perpetrator. The patients themselves have not been able to hold these parts of themselves together in their minds and so the split easily becomes externalized into the environments of forensic services. Typically, conflict within the nursing group gets organized around hard and soft; that is, the hard matter of security and the soft matter of care. These are corollaries to the hard matter of perpetration and the soft matter of victimization.

Because the victim and perpetrator parts of the patient are inevitably split in the patient's mind and indeed often reflected in the structure and organization of services, it may be unsurprising to find that nursing teams tasked with providing care within secure conditions for mentally disordered offenders also find themselves split. However, more than just splitting occurs. The dynamics of difference operate in these environments where hard, security-oriented nurses project their sensitivity and compassion onto and into 'soft' caring nurses who in turn project their sadism and caution into their 'harder' colleagues. Clarke (1996) undertook a covert participant observation into a secure forensic unit and found a typical split within the nursing team; that is, between 'carers' and 'controllers' (p.38). Clarke (1996) as part of his research was able to analyse the relationship between carers and controllers within the forensic unit under study. In keeping with paranoid-schizoid functioning, the controllers in Clarke's study were prone to action rather than thought and were not only hostile towards their thoughtful carer colleagues but were also dismissive of care, undermining the staff support group for example. The caring group of nurses in Clarke's study appeared to find their controlling colleagues disturbing but were nevertheless able to consider their own role in maintaining the split. Clarke's (1996) research identifies one of the key problems in forensic nursing services, which is that as long as such vast splits exist, there is a likelihood that one 'tribe' will never entertain the perspective of the more thinking other. This raises the issue of whether nurses should develop the self-awareness skills necessary to work as professional carers in challenging, emotionally stressful organizations during their pre-registration training (Bray 1998). What seems clear is that in order to address tribal warfare within professional groups in forensic services, support and supervision must be provided to a degree that enables staff to contain the powerful and distressing emotional phenomena projected into them by the patients (Cox 1996). This phenomenon gets organized around difference and the more visible the difference, the more accessible is the target for setting up sado-masochistic relationships which are usually disguised as expressions of legitimate concern.

CONCLUSION

The psychopathology of forensic patients involves the mobilization of primitive defences against anxiety. Nurses who work in close proximity to the patients risk operating in paranoid-schizoid mode too. Exposed to raw, unprocessed projections organized around the victim/perpetrator split in the first instance, nurses are vulnerable to acting out these dynamics and engaging in sado-masochistic functioning if not provided with opportunities to understand the unconscious processes that support this sort of painful interpersonal relating.

In addition to understanding unconscious processes, nurses require supportive, containing structures where they can think about their relationships, test reality and reflect on their experiences thoughtfully. Increased self-awareness can be developed by integrating reflective spaces such as supervision, staff support or experiential groups into nurses' day-to-day working practice. Through these, the ubiquity of projection and the tendency to offload unwanted parts of the self onto others when under emotional pressure can be explored and contained. By recognizing that vulnerability and sadism exists within all of us and can and will be externalized within our relationships from time to time, teams are less likely to organize themselves into victims and perpetrators.

When the unconscious is searching for a receptacle within which to deposit the alien, unwanted part of the self, difference provides an appealing container. This dynamic is inherent within the human condition. However, the more psychologically refined a person is, the less likely to resort to the kind of primitive functioning that supports, for example, racist, sexist or homophobic behaviour one might imagine them to be. People who would not normally feel capable of inflicting pain or humiliation on others or of being regularly bullied, harassed or belittled, can be surprised to find themselves caught up in such intense interpersonal conflict within the forensic workplace. Suddenly feeling oneself to be in a shocking kind of no man's land, is one of the emotionally difficult phenomena that characterises forensic work.

Increased paranoid-schizoid functioning occurs when people are highly anxious or frightened. Nurses working in close proximity to disturbed forensic patients are exposed to milieux that are frequently riddled with anxiety and fear. All people within these environments are prone to paranoid-schizoid functioning, particularly when involved in the management of violent incidents. It is perhaps during the anticipation and aftermath of violence that severe sado-masochistic relating which assumes the form of discriminatory thinking and behaviour is most likely to occur.

An important twist to be observed in the dynamics of difference within forensic services is that victims can also be oppressors because the dynamics underpinning the way people relate are ever present. Unconsciously, the quest to eradicate discrimination can all too often serve as a vessel for sadism. It is for these reasons that promulgation of a culture of enquiry where relationships between staff and patients can be safely explored within containing structures is critical if forensic services are ever to produce lasting change with regard to the difficult atmospheres that have come to define them. That is, change needs to occur below the surface of organizations as well as on top of it and, as such, safely exploring and containing the dynamics of difference would greatly assist the process.

REFERENCES

Bion, W. (1959) 'Attacks on linking.' *International Journal of Psychoanalysis 38*, 266–75.

Bird, J. and Clarke, S. (1999) 'Racism, hatred and discrimination through the lens of projective identification.' *Journal of the Psychonalysis of Culture and Society 4*, 158–61.

Bray, J. (1998) 'Psychiatric Nursing and the Myth of Altruism.' In Barker, P.J. and Davidson, B. (eds) *Psychiatric Nursing and Ethical Strife.* London: Arnold.

Clarke, L. (1996) 'Covert participant observation in a secure forensic unit.' *Nursing Times 92*, 48, 37–40.

Clarke, S. (1999) 'Splitting difference: psychoanalysis, hatred and exclusion.' *Journal for the Theory of Social Behaviour 29*, 1, 21–35.

Cox, M. (1996) 'Psychodynamics and the Special Hospital: "Road Blocks and Thought Blocks".' In Cordess, C. and Cox, M. (eds) *Forensic Psychotherapy: Psychodynamics and the Offender Patient.* 2 vols. London: Jessica Kingsley Publishers.

Dalal, F. (2002) *Race, Colour and the Process of Racialization: New Perspectives from Group Analysis and Sociology.* London: Brunner-Routledge.

Department of Health (1992) *Report of the Committee of Inquiry into Complaints about Ashworth Hospital.* London: HMSO.

Department of Health (2003) *The Independent Inquiry into the Death of David Bennett.* Cambridge: Norfolk, Suffolk and Cambridgeshire Strategic Health Authority.

Fanon, F. (1952) *Black Face: White Masks.* London: Pluto.

Frosh, S. (2005) *Hate and the 'Jewish Science': Anti-Semitism, Nazism and Psychoanalysis.* Basingstoke: Palgrave.

Griffiths, P. and Leach, G. (1998) 'Psychosocial Nursing: A Model Learnt from Experience.' In Barnes, E., Griffiths, P., Ord, J. and Wells, D. (eds) *Face to Face with Distress: The Professional Use of Self in Psychosocial Care.* Oxford: Butterworth-Heinemann.

Horwitz, L. (1983) 'Projective identification in dyads and groups.' *International Journal of Group Psychotherapy 33*, 3, 259–79.

Klein, M. (1946) 'Notes on Some Schizoid Mechanisms.' In M. Klein, *Envy and Gratitude and Other Works, 1946–1963.* London: Hogarth Press and Institute of Psycho-Analysis, 1975.

Menzies Lyth, I. (1988) *Containing Anxiety In Institutions.* London: Free Association Books.

Obholzer, A. (1994) 'Managing Social Anxieties in Public Sector Organizations.' In Obholzer, A. and Roberts, V.Z. (eds) *The Unconscious at Work: Individual and Organizational Stress in the Human Services.* London: Routledge.

SHSA (Special Hospitals Services Authority) (1993) *Report of the Committee of Inquiry into the Death in Broadmoor of Orville Blackwood and a Review of the Deaths of Two Other Afro-Caribbean Patients: 'Big, Black and Dangerous'.* London: SHSA.

Temple, N. (1996) 'Transference and Countertransference: General and Forensic Aspects.' In Cordess, C. and Cox, M. (eds) *Forensic Psychotherapy: Crime, Psychodynamics and the Offender Patient.* 2 vols. London: Jessica Kingsley Publishers.

CHAPTER 6

Paranoid-Schizoid Functioning within a Forensic Intensive Care Ward

Valerie Anne Brown

INTRODUCTION

In this chapter I will explore some of the psychodynamic concepts that help me to understand the emotional environment of the secure mental health setting I work in. I will explain how an understanding of these unconscious processes, which are derived from the Kleinian model of the paranoid-schizoid position, supports my clinical nursing practice. The ward is designated for the intensive care and treatment of people who have a forensic background in that many of the patients have been convicted of unlawful acts of violence against others. Some of the patients have engaged in violence towards staff in mental health settings but have never been charged or convicted. The patients have primary psychiatric diagnoses of severe and often treatment-resistant mental illnesses, such as schizophrenia. For these patients, their severe illnesses occur in the context of a more complex picture, usually involving secondary diagnoses of personality disorders along with a range of other mental health problems. Other patients have primary diagnoses of severe personality disorders, again complicated by a range of other mental health problems, including psychosis. All of the patients on this ward present with behavioural disturbance.

SPLITTING, INTROJECTION, PROJECTION AND THE PARANOID-SCHIZOID POSITION

The first psychodynamic concepts I will describe are projection and introjection. I will consider these concepts together because they form a central part of day-to-day interactions between patients and nurses on the ward. Klein (1997) described the processes of introjection and projection, which she had developed as a result of her psychoanalytic observations of infants and young children. Klein observed that, from the beginning of life, the infant engages in introjection and projection, which are among the earliest activities of the developing mind. Through introjection, the infant takes into himself the persons, relationships and situations that occur within his environment. Eventually, these objects and situations become part of the infant's internal world and inner life. Simultaneously, the infant is able to attribute some of his own internal emotional experiences to other people within his external world. This internal experience usually consists of feelings of love and hate which cannot be held together in the infant's developing mind. Therefore, these feelings are split off and one of them, usually hate, is expelled from the self and attributed to somebody else in the environment. More often than not, in the case of a very young infant, this is the mother. The process of expelling unwanted feelings from the self and attributing them to others is called projection and it takes place to an intense degree during the earliest phase of early development, which Klein (1997) called 'the paranoid-schizoid position'.

According to Klein (1997), with good enough early care, the infant progresses from purely paranoid-schizoid functioning. This occurs when the young mind is able to tolerate feelings of anxiety and guilt about his hateful feelings toward his mother and understand that they occur alongside love in an integrated way. This more mature stage of development was called 'the depressive position' by Klein. At times of stress, for example, people of any age tend to fall back on paranoid-schizoid functioning. Klein described how the paranoid-schizoid functioning served as a fixation point for the development of psychosis later in life. That is, people who suffer from psychotic illnesses operate predominately in the paranoid-schizoid position.

Bion (1970) extended Kleinian theory to groups and placed unconscious processes of projection central to group life. Bion's theory is concerned with the distribution of mental energy within a group and distinguishes two main types of group functioning. The first is the work group which operates in the depressive position (Klein 1997). In the work group energy is concentrated on the task at hand. The work group is able to respond effectively to ever-changing pressures from the environment. Also, the work group is able to constructively address the problems individuals have in working cooperatively with each other. The second type of group described by Bion (1970) operates in paranoid-schizoid mode and is called 'the basic assumption group'. This group feels threatened. As a result, anxiety leads to energy being withdrawn from dealing with the task. This energy is then used to defend the group against its anxieties. Because mental activity is consumed in these defences, no work can be done and no development can occur.

Menzies Lyth (1959), in her now classic work about defensive processes in human services, applied Kleinian theory to the study of organizations. She describes how the powerful paranoid-schizoid defence system which also involves fragmentation and denial of reality can operate at an organizational level, preventing true insights into problems from being gained. Obholzer (1994) describes how, in his work as consulting psychoanalyst to human services, he is struck by way the same unconscious processes that are present in the individual person also operate at an organizational level. De Board (1978) also explains how the same defences against anxiety that shape individual functioning also shape social life in organizations.

In my experience, paranoid-schizoid functioning is ever present in a secure ward for people with challenging behaviours. This exposes nurses who work in close contact with the patients to high levels of projections, usually of intense persecutory anxieties. The extent of these projections is such that even trying to process what belongs to you and what is a projection can be an exhausting task.

Clinical example 1

John is a man in his early thirties who has a primary psychiatric diagnosis of schizophrenia which is treatment resistant. He also has a developmental disorder which makes it difficult for him to tolerate unstructured, unpredictable events. John spends a lot of his time in seclusion as a result of repeated violent assaults on nurses. John has remained extremely violent for many years and has caused significant injury to nursing staff in the recent past. He is six feet, six inches tall and well built, yet perceives himself to be at risk from everyone around him. When nursing staff engage with John, they report overwhelming feelings of fear and anxiety. The question they struggle with is: whose fear and anxiety is it? On the one hand nurses have been physically injured by John on a fairly regular basis so it is understandable that they would feel as they do. On the other hand, it is equally possible that John locates his own dangerousness onto the nurses: is what they feel a projection of his fear and anxiety about what they might do to him?

John's feelings and thoughts are experienced by him in a concrete way. Sohn (1999) has explained how the person suffering from psychosis tends to operate concretely because their capacity for symbol formation is absent. Therefore, unable to distinguish between one's own mind and that of the other, in psychosis, the patient engages in physical acts to resolve feelings that otherwise would be regarded as depressive anxiety. In John's case, this means that if he feels unsafe, the only solution available to him is to force others, through physical actions, to make him safe, also by applying a physical solution. John is not able to distinguish where this lack of safety originates from in terms of self or the object. He is not able to recognize whether danger has its roots internally from the self or externally from nursing staff. This dynamic is paralleled in the nurses who do not know whether their fear emanates from within themselves or from John. Nurses who engage interpersonally with John are required to be both container and contained, to use Bion's terms. They need to provide John with psychological containment, by thinking about their emotional experiences rather than acting out (for example by fight or flight) on them, as to do so would risk John feeling uncontained, which in turn would result in violent behaviour as he became overwhelmed with fear and anxiety.

Developmental history

To better understand John's pattern of interpersonal relating, it is important to understand his developmental history. He was born into a single parent family and does not know who his father is, being conceived when his mother was studying abroad. His mother had three other children by different fathers. John has an older sister and a younger brother. A third sibling died soon after birth. John was placed in foster care from soon after birth until he was three years old. He was placed in foster care by his mother who did not feel she had the capacity to care for another child at that time and wanted to continue to pursue her studies. John was placed in a number of foster placements during the first three years of his life. At least one set of foster parents were found to have profoundly deprived John of emotional and physical care, leading to delays in reaching his developmental milestones, especially speech. Although John's mother later undertook to provide him with a home, the damage had apparently been done. He became a very disturbed child, requiring psychiatric treatment from the age of seven. He spent his childhood and adolescence in continual residential care, moving from placement to placement due to disturbed behaviour and violence. He was admitted to a secure mental health service following repeated assaults on care workers in a secure social services placement.

Assaultive behaviour

One afternoon on the ward, I informed John, who was in seclusion, that his mother had contacted the ward to say that she and John's younger brother had returned home from their holiday abroad. I informed John that his mother had requested to speak to him. I relayed this message to John without predicting any problems and suggested he might like to phone his family.

Later that afternoon the nurses took John's meal to him in his room at which time he appeared calm and spoke of phoning his mother during the evening. When nurses opened the door to his room, he rapidly jumped to his feet and attempted to assault one of them. A violent incident took place in John's room and physical injury was only narrowly prevented.

Following the incident, nurses were able to reflect on what happened. We concluded that the violent assault occurred for two main reasons: first, John's envy and jealousy regarding his mother and sibling going on holiday together and, second, the nurses had not only reminded him of his feelings about his mother but had also threatened to disturb him, taking him from the safety of his room. That made his anxiety reach such a pitch that it amounted to significant psychic pain. As Bell (2000) says, a severe form of tormenting psychic pain can arise from feelings of being persecuted internally by the lingering complaints of internalized psychic objects. This level of psychic pain can, according to Bell, lead to acts of severe violence that can be considered as murderousness and may be either internally or externally directed in an effort to be rid of such unbearable mental anguish.

John dealt with his overwhelming, unbearable feelings by resorting to physically violent acts because, as a result of his illness, he was not able to process those difficult feelings through thought. Concretely, his murderousness was directed at trying to kill his pain and what he perceived to be the source of that pain, the nurses. During the violent behaviour John appeared out of control as he tried by any means available to destroy the nurses in front of him. He kicked, hit out with his fists and attempted to bite nurses when restrained. Throughout the incident he was screaming obscenities usually reserved for his mother when, for example, she fails to turn up for a planned visit. He called the nurses whores and prostitutes. I believe at that moment, in John's mind all the nurses present in that room were his mother, a truly disturbing thought. John's inability to symbolize meant there was no 'as if' quality to his transference feelings so the nurses became the mother who in his infancy threatened his survival by abandonment, neglect and deprivation. News of her return from holiday with his younger sibling stirred up these feelings. Also, his rage and terror were projected and attacked in a self-preservative way. The result was that he needed to be contained both physically and psychologically.

Reflection

In trying to fully understand why John reacted as he did to his mother's return from holiday and the request that he phone her, it was important that nurses reflect on why we had not predicted that his reaction would have been a violent one. For example, I had not remembered his ambivalent feelings toward his mother.

There were other nurses on duty at the time who also failed to make that link so I do not claim sole responsibility for 'forgetting' about his complicated relationship with his mother. Most of the nurses were able to reflect that being told of the phone call had not only stimulated John, it had forced him to make contact with thoughts and feelings he had no wish to experience. Consciously and unconsciously he had been disturbed and experienced no other possible outlet but violence.

Dynamics within the nursing team

It is arguably the extent of John's murderousness that makes the nursing staff tasked with caring for him feel vulnerable. However, there is a split in attitudes within the nursing team. At one end of the spectrum, some nurses feel that we are working with a deeply disturbed and dangerous man and so we must be prepared for any violence at all times. At the other end of the spectrum, there are nurses who mostly see the victim in John, that is, the ill person who is not responsible for his actions. Neither of these extreme positions is healthy for John or the team and reflective practice enables nursing staff to work through their counter-transference feelings.

Further splitting is present on a day-by-day basis surrounding decisions to engage with John and the degree of physical containment required to do so. As nurses it feels uncomfortable to know that we are not physically able to restrain a patient without recourse to support from other clinical areas within the service. As a result this position can lead to inaction if it is felt unsafe to enter John's seclusion room, leaving him increasingly isolated and to all intents and purposes recreating the deprivation he experienced as an infant. At the other extreme there are nurses who believe that he can be managed without excessive risk regardless of his level of arousal. However well meaning the latter strategy is, this does not make John feel contained and his anxiety along with concomitant projections increase accordingly. It is, however, possible to predict whether John is at high risk of assaulting other people by making behavioural observations. Physical signs of his distress and related risk can be assessed by the presence of sweating, shaking, pressure of speech and hyperventilation. However, it can be a challenge to convince nurses of the reliability of these risk factors when they themselves are overwhelmed with fear and anxiety when in contact with John. The task of maintaining a therapeutic relationship with John is a very delicate one and requires nursing staff to make sophisticated clinical judgements about his mental state and risk. The dilemma facing nurses working with John is similar to Fonagy's (2003) observation about the way mothers regulate their babies' emotional states. If nurses, unable to contain the projections, reflect back to John the emotional state he is experiencing, such as fear or anger, his own emotional state is likely to deteriorate and the associated risk of violence will increase. This describes well the concerns that the nurses have about their communications with John.

Splitting is also manifest in the way a person divides up the good and bad feelings which are about the same individual and attributes them to separate people, often resulting in conflict between the 'good' and 'bad' factions. John relates to the nurses who mostly experience him as ill and not responsible for his actions as though they are all good. He relates to the nurses who experience him as dangerous and sadistic as though they are all bad. The function of this splitting for John is that he does not have to negotiate painful thoughts about other people or indeed himself. By experiencing other people as all good or all bad, he does not have to integrate within his mind the fact that even good people will let him down or get things wrong about his care. Likewise, he does not need to feel guilt about having hateful feelings about people who are sometimes helpful towards him and who look after him. This is an example of paranoid-schizoid functioning and the danger is that the environment comes to reflect the deep split in John's internal world. Nurses holding vastly different views about him are prone to engage in professional conflicts about how best to care for him safely. Reflective practice and supervision groups provide a safe, containing space where nurses can think about these dynamics with the aim of integrating something of the patient's internal life that he cannot manage to achieve by himself.

Splitting in the nursing team

The intensive care ward operates a system of internal rotation. This means that individual nurses work both day and night shifts on a rotational basis. The difference between day and night shifts at any given time can provide an opportunity for splitting within the ward. For patients functioning in paranoid-schizoid mode, it is difficult to maintain ambivalent feelings for both groups of nurses and so the tendency is to split them into, for example, good day staff and bad night staff. When patients suffer severe psychopathology, this splitting can be dangerous.

Clinical example 2

Mark has a primary psychiatric diagnosis of bipolar disorder and secondary diagnoses of borderline and antisocial personality disorders. He has a personal history of early abandonment by his mother and spent many years in residential care as a child where he was the victim of sexual abuse. He has spent most of his adult life in secure institutions where he has engaged in violent behaviour towards others, mainly nurses. In the past he has been convicted of attempted murder following an offence where he tried to strangle a prison officer while on remand.

Mark's behaviour on the ward differs depending on whether it is day time or night time. During the day Mark usually engages well with the ward programme and gets along well with the nurses. He struggles with his desire to do well in this placement with his good intentions often undermined by his unstable mood. Nurses are able to identify when Mark is at risk of behaving in ways that are unsafe because he experiences physiological changes that are observable: for example, when Mark becomes elated his pupils dilate. These observable changes enable nurses to work proactively with Mark and he is amenable to collaborative working to manage his instability of mood. As a result, he is able to avoid tipping into episodes of behavioural disturbance that have in the past concluded with acts of violence and self-injury.

During the night, Mark is not so able to manage his affective problems. He often gets involved in arguments with nurses, denies he has any mental health problems and seeks collusive relationships with nurses who often feel pressurized to agree with him that he no longer needs psychiatric medication. Mark is frequently hostile towards night nursing staff. This is the case even if the night nursing staff had recently been working days where they had been able to work collaboratively with Mark. Nursing staff who have had this experience report that they feel as though Mark regards them as two separate people. They feel as though they were one person while working with him during the day and a different person entirely when undertaking night duty.

Mark's projections are experienced by nurses as powerful and night nursing staff report strong urges to go home when Mark confronts them in angry, combative ways. Many of the night nurses feel that Mark expresses his murderousness when challenging them about house rules and as a result they find it difficult to maintain ward, professional and interpersonal boundaries. Mark's hostility is such that night nurses feel that he is communicating that they either do as he says or else he will kill them.

In order to gain a better understanding of what might be going on between Mark and the night nursing staff when they feel as though he is threatening their lives it is useful to know a little more about his personal history of trauma. Mark has a history of prolonged, sadistic, sexual abuse that was perpetrated during his childhood. This abuse occurred over a number of years when he was placed in a residential children's home. The perpetrator was a teacher at the school and Mark was threatened with death if he did not comply with the teacher's demands. As an abandoned child, he was vulnerable and felt that he had nobody to turn to. On the ward, nurses on the receiving end of Mark's demands that they agree with his point of view or do what he wants them to do in terms of transgressing house rules, experience something of the emotional intensity of the abusive relationship Mark had as a child with his teacher. Zachary (1997) has described how the murderous forensic patient needs to have such feelings contained until they are able to recognize their identification with their original abuser. Zachary was referring to the function of forensic psychotherapists working with murderous patients. However, it may be argued that in their interactions with Mark, night nurses on the ward are required to contain his murderousness.

The dynamics of Mark's relationships with the night nurses involve splitting, projection, traumatic re-enactment and identification with the aggressor (Freud 1946). It is possible that, for this patient, night time in hospital stirs up horrors relating to his abuse in childhood by a professional carer. However, he has identified with this abuser and attempts to terrorize and coerce nursing staff into corrupting and transgressing boundaries, much as his abuser did in order to violate the boundaries of Mark's body and of the caring relationship. The nurses' task is to stand their ground with Mark in the face of the onslaught of hostility and projections, and remain within their professional roles. Being in a position to think about the dynamics of the situation helps them to achieve this. Nevertheless, the nurses' task is a difficult one to achieve and the emotional impact of this work is immense. For that reason, the split between day and night nursing teams must be recognized and addressed. Otherwise, relationships between the two nursing groups are likely to become very disturbed.

One further hypothesis about why Mark splits the day and night nursing teams into good and bad camps is that his abuser may have been experienced by him, as a child, as two separate people. In other words, the abuser may have presented as a kindly, helpful teacher during the day time and a violent, ruthless rapist at night. Adding some weight to this hypothesis is the way Mark refers to the night nurses. He always calls the night staff 'they' when he discusses their 'cruelty' and complains about how badly he has been treated. He never refers to any of the night nursing staff by name, as though they were strangers. The danger for the staff team is of the two groups of nurses remaining separate and not coming together to think about Mark and their relationships with him. By meeting together in a group reflective space, it is possible to develop a working hypothesis about the dynamics in operation, together as a team. If this does not happen, there becomes a high possibility of the split created by Mark being acted out within the nursing team. In all probability, day staff would attribute the difficulties to mismanagement of Marks' care by the night nurses. Simultaneously, night nursing staff would put Mark's settled behaviour during the day down to day nurses colluding with him and transgressing ward boundaries and house rules. If a situation such as this arises, conflict will be acted out within the ward nursing team. It is the task of forensic clinicians to understand the violent person's psychic reality, not just in order to be able to offer treatment, but also to better predict the nature of the risk presented both to themselves and to others (Cox 1982).

CONCLUSION

It may be inappropriate to offer psychodynamic psychotherapy to forensic patients who have the most severe psychopathologies and whose murderous rage and challenging behaviours present a significant risk of harm. However, a psychodynamic perspective integrated with forensic nursing practice can be helpful in terms of providing a way to understand much of the disturbance that takes place within secure mental health services. In particular, the paranoid-schizoid position can provide a viable model for understanding primitive psychological functioning at the level of the individual, the team and the organization.

REFERENCES

Bell, D. (2000) 'Who is killing what or whom? Some notes on the internal phenomenology of suicide.' *Psychoanalytic Psychotherapy 15*, 1, 21–37.

Bion, W.R. (1970) *Attention and Interpretation. A Scientific Approach to Insight in Psycho-Analysis and Groups.* London: Tavistock.

Cox, M. (1982) 'The Psychotherapist as Assessor of Dangerousness.' In Hamilton, J.R. and Freeman, H. (eds) *Dangerousness: Psychiatric Assessment and Management.* London: Gaskell.

De Board, R. (1978) *The Psychoanalysis of Organizations.* London: Routledge.

Fonagy, P. (2003) 'The Developmental Roots of Violence in the Failure of Mentalization.' In Pfäfflin, F. and Adshead, G. (eds) *A Matter of Security: The Application of Attachment Theory to Forensic Psychiatry and Psychotherapy.* London: Jessica Kingsley Publishers.

Freud, A. (1946) *The Ego and the Mechanisms of Defence.* New York: International Universities Press.

Klein, M. (1997) *Envy and Gratitude and Other Works, 1946–1963.* London: Vintage.

Menzies Lyth (1959) 'The Functioning of Social Systems as a Defence against Anxiety: A Report on a Study of the Nursing Service of a General Hospital.' In *Containing Anxiety in Institutions. Selected Essays,* Volume 1. London: Free Association Books, 1988.

Obholzer, A. (1994) 'Managing Social Anxieties in Public Sector Organizations.' In Obholzer, A. and Roberts, V.Z. (eds) *The Unconscious at Work: Individual and Organizational Stress in the Human Services.* London: Routlege.

Sohn, L. (1999) 'Psychosis and Violence.' In Williams, P. (ed.) *Psychosis (Madness) (Psychoanalytic Ideas).* London: Karnac.

Zachary, A. (1997) 'Murderousness.' In Welldon, E.V. and Van Velsen, C. (eds) *A Practical Guide to Forensic Psychotherapy.* Part 2. London: Jessica Kingsley Publishers.

CHAPTER 7

Reflecting on Murderousness: Reflective Practice in Secure Forensic Settings

Stephen Mackie

INTRODUCTION

In this chapter I wish to consider some aspects that are involved in weekly ongoing staff support groups in forensic secure settings. I will attempt to describe their usefulness and the form of support they can provide as well as exploring aspects that can make them difficult for both the members of the group and the facilitator. Many different and diverse issues arise in ward reflective practice groups but perhaps the most difficult to explore is that of destructiveness and murderousness, aspects that inevitably percolate throughout a secure forensic service as a result of its containment of violent, psychotic offenders.

There are numerous, seemingly interchangeable, terms for this kind of work in psychiatric institutions. This runs the risk of blurring and creating confusion in knowing what the true task of the various structures are. In mental health nursing the term 'clinical supervision' has been adopted to describe the professional and managerial supervision structures and 'staff support' is often adopted to describe the structures developed around debriefings following serious untoward incidents where staff or the organization have been traumatized in some way. I will therefore use the term 'reflective practice' in order to differentiate ongoing and regular support that is offered to wards using psychodynamic thinking from these other structures, the aim being to discuss, explore and understand emotional aspects and issues that are involved in the experience of being a nurse on a particular clinical area or ward. Reflective practice also offers a space where curiosity can develop.

THE PROJECTION OF PSYCHOTIC ANXIETIES

A forensic psychiatric ward or institution is often a maelstrom of psychotic anxieties, split off from the patient's mind and violently projected out. These extremely toxic agents, evacuated by mentally ill offenders, spread throughout the institutional space that is designed to contain them. These institutions utilize three main methods in order to fulfil their task of providing the containment of dangerous and disturbing anxiety:

1. A concrete containment provided by the bricks, mortar, windows, doors and fences of the institution.
2. A chemical containment provided by medication, managing the intensity of disturbing anxiety in patients.
3. An emotional containment provided by the minds of those in contact with these patients.

As nursing staff, more than any other discipline (apart, perhaps, from health care assistants), are in close emotional contact with patients 24 hours a day, seven days weeks, violent, psychotic projections inevitably invade the minds of these people, contaminating their thinking, feelings and behaviour. They are exposed to a constant, high level of emotional disturbance. Reflective practice groups of the type I have in mind may be able to help staff tolerate their exposure to these 'toxins' and understand them in a way that can be beneficial to the growth and development of both the nurses and their patients. The potential psychological containment provided by a reflective practice group is what I wish to focus upon.

THE CONTAINING FUNCTION

The concept of 'containment' was conceptualized by Bion (1962) and summarized by Segal:

> When an infant has an intolerable anxiety, he deals with it by projecting it into the mother. The mother's response is to acknowledge the anxiety and do whatever is necessary to relieve the infant's distress. The infant's perception is that he has projected something intolerable into his object, but the object was capable of containing and dealing with it. He can then re-introject not only his original anxiety but an anxiety modified by it having been contained. He also introjects an object capable of containing and dealing with anxiety. The containment of anxiety by an external object capable of understanding is the beginning of mental stability. (Segal 1975, p.134)

Bion believed that emotional contact could be thought about as a process of containing.

THE ROLE OF THE FORENSIC MENTAL HEALTH NURSE

I now wish to diverge briefly in order to describe my view of the therapeutic role of a forensic mental health nurse. It is a containing role and encompasses both care-taking and potent functions. Care-taking is the task that nurses undertake in order to provide safe, stable and supportive environments and relationships that may enable patients to feel sufficiently secure in order that they may be able to tolerate being introduced to 'doses' of reality by the nursing team (the potent function). This might be, for example, the basic but fundamental reality that they are patients receiving treatment within a hospital and that they have needs. The psychotic aspect of a patient (as differentiated from a more healthy aspect of a patient's mind) cannot tolerate awareness of normal human needs, vulnerabilities and dependency and wishes to attack and kill off awareness of this reality by attacking the perception, or the source of awareness of reality (Bion 1957). In practice, therefore, there can be considerable fear created in both patients and staff around confronting patients with reality; the fear being of the eruption of explosive violence. The anxiety inherent in the work of a forensic mental health nurse can be particularly intense as many of their patients do not just have the wish to kill off reality but have, in truth, actually killed or attacked the source of the awareness of reality, their victims. They have similarly attacked another source of awareness of reality: their own minds.

Returning to the containing function, Segal continues:

> This mental stability may be disrupted from two sources. The mother may be unable to bear the infant's projected anxiety and he (the infant) may introject an experience of even greater terror than the one he had projected. It may also be disrupted by excessive destructive omnipotence of the infant's phantasy. (Segal 1975, p.135)

The inability of a nursing team to tolerate their patient's projections (an inability to tolerate their patients and their disturbance) therefore increases the anxiety of their patients and so can feed an escalating cycle of disturbance and breakdown, with the potential for the eruption of violence.

In order to contain their patients' anxieties, and therefore their violence, nurses need to be able to both experience and tolerate the anxiety created by contact with this type of patient. That is, they need to be able to tolerate their patient's often violent projections. For example, it is very important that staff can, at times, feel frightened by their patients. To feel robust enough to engage in this kind of work nursing staff themselves need to feel sufficiently contained and secure. As with their patients, they must feel that there are secure, stable and supportive structures around them.

A number of factors can contribute to a reduction in the ability of nurses to tolerate these projections:

1. External demands may reduce nurses' capacities to undertake this containing function, for example budgetary requirements alongside the current culture of government initiatives that demand nurses' attention away from their patients and their clinical work.
2. Internal, personal experiences, perhaps anger or frustration about work or personal relationships, produce additional demands for attention and will undermine the capacity to cope with demands placed upon nurses by their patients.
3. Insufficient resources: for example, staff shortages, environmental structures that do not feel safe, professional structures that do not feel supportive and no longer feeling kept in the minds of one's clinical colleagues. Also, aspects that are central to a mental health nurse's identity – empathy, emotional

> understanding and caring – are not just attacked in phantasy by patients, but can become unfashionable, looked down on in a modern health culture of intellectualized learning, evidence-based practice and measurable outcomes. They are difficult to measure scientifically and therefore seemingly difficult to defend and justify.

When any or a combination of the three above factors is severe enough, difficulties can arise. This interpolation of too great internal and/or external pressures with insufficient resources often mirrors the explosive mixture that combined to create the circumstances where a patient's tragic index offence occurred.

COLLECTIVE DEFENCES

Without adequate support and when patients' projections can no longer be borne or contained by the nursing team a number of defensive measures will arise. As Menzies Lyth (1960) stated in her paper exploring defensive structures used by nurses in a training hospital, the main aim of the staff becomes that of self-preservation rather than that of helping the patient. In other words, under intense pressure of anxiety the main task of the nursing team now becomes the relief from anxiety. Hinshelwood (1979) describes a collective evasion of the experience of anxiety in preference to facing it and working with it in order to achieve some maturation. He points out that this evasion inevitably leads to a reciprocal detachment from oneself, one's professional and personal identity and often leads to a sense of emptiness and of having nothing valuable to offer:

> In the course of time such uncertainty eats into the confidence of the staff collectively. They may begin to lose sight of their own roles and purpose and their sense of value to the institution. Eventually they will look around for roles which they feel will enhance the sense of adequacy and value and in turn they feel encroached on by others who are also looking round. Friction and this special form of rivalry come to the fore, the staff seem no longer to be working for the collective purpose of the institution but rather for themselves, to find their own feet in their jobs as they feel the foundation of their self-esteem slipping away from under them. (Hinshelwood 1979, p.90)

In extreme cases, this can be seen in wards where staff experience the need to avoid any real emotional contact with their patients as this is felt to be too threatening. Staff may spend much time in their nursing station while patients reciprocally spend much time in their own rooms. An empty, lifeless ward atmosphere may confront the visitor. Unfortunately, the price paid by nurses for this 'peaceful arrangement' is the disavowing of reality themselves. They now exist in an anxiety-free but deadened environment where no one appears troubled but creativity and life have been killed off. Neither staff nor patients are able to develop in any real way. The ability to obtain and receive real help has also become a casualty of this defensive arrangement.

AIMS OF REFLECTIVE PRACTICE

In order to be effective in and to gain satisfaction from our work and obtain a personal sense of satisfaction and meaning from what we do, we need to feel emotionally involved: with our patients, our work, our profession and ourselves. We need to attempt to understand our own anxieties and difficulties as well as our patients' in order to prevent a defensive distancing from our patients and so ourselves.

Within a psychodynamic frame, the use of individual, team or ward reflective practice is one method of supporting and helping nurses tolerate difficult emotions and experiences resulting from providing interpersonal care to patients, the aim being to create a reflective space, protected from intrusions of normal daily routine and structures, whereby an understanding of staff's anxieties and the source of these anxieties can be attempted. Our anxiety becomes more tolerable and manageable when it is better understood, that is, thought about. This also allows us to tolerate and understand our patients' states of mind more effectively, to empathize and so contain their anxieties and projections better.

As one of the aims of the psychotic aspects of the personality is to attack this thinking and awareness, I will describe two examples of the use and dynamics of regular once-weekly reflective practice groups for nurses on two different secure forensic wards.

Case example: Thinking and the wish not to think

A ward had been extremely disturbed for a long period with regular outbursts of violence between patients and towards staff. In response to this many of the more disturbed patients were distributed throughout other wards in order to reduce the intensity of the violence in this one clinical area. After the ward was more settled the nursing team requested support and were offered once-weekly ongoing reflective practice.

In the early days of the reflective practice group the nursing team talked of how they put on psychological armour when they came to work in order to survive each shift, taking it off again once they left. They also, in the initial meetings, came to the reflective practice group wearing this armour and so were able to bring their problem directly into the group so it may be reflected upon and therefore thought about.

After some time of cautious discussion and exploration a nurse exclaimed, 'I'm like a crack addict. I feel very uncomfortable when the ward is settled, I feel lost. I don't know what is going on. I want to get busy again.' Another member agreed: 'I feel I must be mad saying this but at least it was clear where the attack was coming from.' I suggested that there may therefore be some investment in the ward being more violent, disturbed and demanding and even, somewhere, a wish for it to be so again in order to avoid confronting something more uncomfortable and disturbing.

Another nurse agreed, 'Yes, you end up thinking when it's settled. I feel guilty that I no longer know what to do as a clinical nurse – it's been so long.' This was at a point where it could be seen that under their armour was also a guarded suspiciousness of my motives. They began to anticipate harsh criticism and judgement from me and, indeed, attempted to subtly provoke me into criticizing or 'attacking' their clinical practice which would support their suspicions that I was there to persecute them.

It now appeared that what was actually persecuting the team was an extremely intolerant and tyrannical guilt, common in the kind of patients found in a forensic establishment. The armour and disturbance defended them from contact with this severe psychotic guilt but it also resulted in a detachment from their own selves. They felt lost and emotionally distant from themselves, their work and their professionalism.

Over time the nurses had adapted to their previously traumatic working conditions. Years of contact with very disturbed patients and their intense persecutory and violent projections had a disturbing, persecutory effect on the nurses and the violent activity meant that there had been little space for the activity of thinking.

With the ward being more settled they had more space to reflect on themselves and their work but were distressed at what they found. They found their behaviour and thinking, or lack of thinking, mirroring that of their patients: a mad addiction to violence and destructiveness that was at odds with their view of themselves. What they were beginning to make emotional contact with and what was becoming more conscious was something within them that had been attacking their own capacities as experienced nurses and clinicians – a severe and tyrannical sense of guilt. They felt that they were becoming the 'patients'. This is when they requested the help of a reflective practice group.

A terribly harsh super-ego had been violently projected into the staff by their patients. It was further projected into me in the group, pressing me to wish to judge them critically. They were communicating to me, in a powerful, non-verbal way, their experience of being on the receiving end of this projection, which had been located into them by their patients. The patients were a population who could not tolerate any guilt that resulted from their acts of aggression, hostility and murderousness.

With time and working through these very difficult issues the team was able to regain contact with their true capacities as experienced clinicians. The work also helped the staff understand more about their patients' addiction to disturbed states of mind as a way of avoiding contact with feelings of guilt and despair.

Case example: An attack on awareness and thinking

In another ward reflective practice group the team presented themselves in one session in a manner that suggested that they did not feel they needed reflective practice but presented a patient case for discussion. This presentation was unusual in that the nurses presented the patient as someone no longer needing their forensic team input. Apparently he was doing well and as the multidisciplinary team did not feel that they could provide a service for him they were considering his transfer to non-secure psychiatric services.

What was unusual was that teams usually bring the issues which are causing them the most anxiety to reflective practice. Therefore, what was it about this patient who presented so well but also caused the most anxiety for the team? It appeared to me that for the team to experience themselves as having any needs was considered threatening and rather than be aware of their need for help they would rather appease me (as being the one with 'needs' at that moment) so that they could, in phantasy, discharge me, get rid of me and get on with business.

Eventually, from the team's discussion, it became clearer that although the patient's care plan was concerned with his moving on, the patient was in reality very fragile. He could not tolerate any contact with reality and this included all those who represented the reality that he was an ill patient who needed help. He managed his world by massively projecting into those around him, including his multidisciplinary team, his psychotic disturbance, including his murderous wishes to kill awareness of reality.

The wish to transfer him to non-secure services was an unconscious collusion with that aspect of the patient who wanted to be seen and to see himself as someone not dangerous. There was pressure to appease him as well as the wish to have this dangerous patient located far away, which was in turn a reflection of the patient's need to split off his dangerousness and locate it far away in others.

One nurse in this reflective practice group found himself lending the patient money. Being a nurse very aware of the importance of boundaries, this was something he would normally be very conscientious about not doing. This is what alerted me to the feeling that there was a tremendous anxiety for those around this patient. The nurses were being forced out of their professional roles as clinical nurses.

It transpired that, to make true contact, both emotionally and physically, with this patient was a very frightening thing to do, especially as those team members represented the reality that this patient hated and he did have the potential to kill anyone who represented that reality. The nurses described the pressure to 'play down' their professional role and be more 'friendly' and appeasing, responding to the pressure expressed by this patient. A nurse recounted the patient telling him, 'I wish you weren't a nurse – I would enjoy being friends with you'. The message being, 'Be my friend, not my foe – I hate you being a nurse who makes me aware of the reality that I am a patient with needs. I wish to kill off any awareness that I may have as well as any awareness that you have in your mind.'

What the nursing team was struggling with mirrored the patient's own internal struggle, that is, the wish to kill and get rid off that which was so disturbing – awareness of reality. The difference was that the nursing team was aware that something was not as it seemed and it did disturb them.

Their disturbance stemmed from their own wishes to kill off the patient symbolically by discharging him and so get rid of that source of disturbance. This was also expressed in the reflective practice group through the wanting to appease and quickly get rid off the facilitator who may actually allow them to make contact with their own thoughts and feelings.

The psychotic murderous aspects of their patient's personality had been forcefully projected into the nurses, attacking and to a degree taking over their minds and their thinking. These aspects also threatened them into colluding with the psychotic parts of the patient and 'agreeing' that he was well. The nursing team's awareness, at some level, of the misfit and discomfort of these ill-sitting projections was what had enabled them to bring this case for reflection and so re-engage with their thinking about this patient.

At some level the nurses were aware of their doubts about the transfer but needed the outside support of a mind that was not contaminated by such close contact with this patient in order to help them clarify and regain contact with their professional minds (selves). The team then felt able to think freely and reconsider the patient's transfer and then discuss their thoughts and feelings with the rest of the multidisciplinary team. It transpired that the patient's consultant had also questioned his own mind about the transfer but hadn't been able to clarify what his doubts were and so considered them unreasonable. The patient's transfer plan was reconsidered.

DIFFICULTIES IN MAKING CONTACT AND POTENTIAL FAILURES OF REFLECTIVE PRACTICE

It is very difficult for clinical staff to think about and so make contact with these destructive and murderous aspects that wish to kill off and get rid of neediness, thinking and knowing. It is disturbing to 'know' that we too can have these phantasies. There is often a wish to 'get rid of' this knowing and ward staff may wish to get rid of the reflective practice group and its facilitator as potential sources of 'knowing'. This can be expressed by a nursing team 'forgetting' each week that their reflective practice session was occuring.

It is not always the contact with their patients that can disturb staff. It is often contact with their own thoughts and feelings that create the greatest anxiety for a team. This is especially so in more acute areas where staff experience a barrage of violent, psychotic projections being put into them, so much so that it can become difficult to differentiate what belongs to whom.

It is important to keep in mind that these are phantasies, often unconscious, and very different from the psychotic murderousness of the patients. This differentiation can become eroded in the minds of staff in contact with these patients, leaving them feeling that they are actually mad and are 'the patients'.

My two clinical examples contain within them examples of potential failures of reflective practice. In the first example the nurses' guilt about murderous phantasies persecuted them so intensely that they wished to avoid any contact with these very difficult feelings by attempting both to avoid attending the support group that they so wanted and to provoke the facilitator to give up on them out of frustration and terminate the relationship with the ward. In both examples there was pressure on the facilitator to presume that the nursing team did not want him or care about their reflective practice, that they had no needs, which could lead to the facilitator feeling useless and dejected and wishing to avoid these uncomfortable experiences (perhaps his own murderous and revengeful impulses) by distancing himself from working with the ward. I would view these experiences in the facilitator as a communication by the team of their own current experiences of feeling useless and dejected and that what they have to offer their patients is constantly attacked and got rid of.

As a potential source of knowing and thinking, a reflective practice group will inevitably be attacked in some way. This dynamic is at the fore in a secure forensic setting, in with the bricks. Indeed it is important that the reflective practice structure can allow itself to be attacked in order that these dynamics can be made available for understanding. Therefore, reflective practice facilitators also need to feel contained, by a combination of their own professional structures and their own internal supportive structures. It is important that they can survive, and be experienced as surviving, the murderous projections that arise in forensic reflective practice groups when they function well. This in itself offers support to the group members by allowing them to experience that their fears and anxieties, often contaminated by their patients' own psychotic anxieties, are not the 'end of the world'. If a facilitator is experienced as breaking down and displaying anxiety himself, turning up late for sessions, frequently cancelling sessions, this can, unconsciously, create concern in the members that their anxieties are too much to tolerate and are dangerous. The collective defences, personal detachment and despair may then increase.

CONCLUSION

Reflective practice works well if it can enable nurses to make contact with their anxiety. They will then be more able to make clinical judgements that are based upon the real needs of patients rather than on a need to avoid anxiety. They will be more able to tolerate the anxieties and stresses of their work without feeling the need to disengage from the emotional contact and the impact of what they are required to process in their work.

Reflective practice provides an alternative to creating defensive detachment from the experience of anxiety. This alternative is to seek a therapeutic way out through facing the experience and working through it rather than evading it. Our concerns, fears, worries, anger, resentment and hate need to be faced and understood within the context of our work with very disturbed patients, in order that we can remain engaged with our work, and gain personal satisfaction and development from that experience. Holding onto defensive structures leads only to a loss of contact with our patients, our profession and with our emotions. We therefore lose contact with ourselves. The aim of this form of support is therefore to try and help nursing staff broaden their spectrum of awareness, thinking and feeling in order to allow them increased freedom to be able to think about their clinical and work issues, how they feel about them and to make decisions based upon that thinking and feeling. Support is therefore obtained through understanding.

REFERENCES

Bion, W. (1957) 'Differentiation of the psychotic from the non-psychotic personalities.' *International Journal of Psychoanalysis 38*, 266–75.

Bion, W. (1962) 'A theory of thinking.' *International Journal of Psychoanalysis 43*, 306–10.

Hinshelwood, R.D. (1979) 'Democratisation in the hospital community.' *Group Analysis 12*, 84–93.

Menzies Lyth, I. (1960) 'The functioning of a social defense system as a defense against anxiety.' *Human Relations 11*, 95–121.

Segal, H. (1975) 'A Psychoanalytic Approach to the Treatment of Psychosis.' In *The Work of Hannah Segal.* New York: Jason Aronson.

CHAPTER 8

Containment and the Structured Day

Sarita Bose

INTRODUCTION

The concept of providing a timetabled day of events and activities for an inpatient setting is by no means a new idea. The mental health nurse training mainly focuses on a holistic model of care, incorporating socio-economic, legal/ethical, humanistic, medical and psychological influences (frequently along a cognitive and behavioural model) to the understanding of the provision of activities and group work for patients. Development of coping skills, the learning of new creative and vocational skills and abilities, social contact, stabilization of mental state and peer support are some of the many benefits of having an active daily programme. However, when providing such activities and routine for forensic psychiatric inpatients, I have found that attempting to provide all of the above to improve those patients' mental states has been at times ineffective and complicated. This may be due to the severity and complexity of their psychopathology, their crimenogenic needs and their propensity to violently acting out aggressive impulses. Therefore in addition to all the above models of care and treatment, in this chapter, it is my intention to apply W.R. Bion's psychodynamic concept of 'psychological containment' to the provision of a structured daily programme of activities for a detained forensic psychiatric population. My discussion will emphasize this theory in relation to its usefulness on admission facilities in any forensic psychiatric hospital.

THE FORENSIC PATIENT

On transfer to any forensic admission unit patients are often very vulnerable, mentally unstable and violent to others and themselves. They may be unable to contain their conscious and unconscious emotions and phantasies of fear, rage, anxiety, insecurity and vulnerability. They often exhibit behaviours that repel, frighten and reject nurses' offers of help and support. Patients often feel out of control of their minds and bodies and are confused by their own behaviour. They are frequently stuck in a repetitive cycle of re-enacting unprocessed childhood traumas. They do not appear to learn from their mistakes. Most powerfully and significantly, forensic patients have come to experience a nurse's (or other mental health professional's) gestures of 'caring' as equivalent to seduction, cruelty and domination, and ultimately as abusive care. The vast majority of the forensic patients I have worked with come to these services with histories of unrelenting trauma and life events, sometimes from birth. These negative developmental antecedents often include a combination of neglect, emotional, physical and sexual abuse, loss or abandonment and inconsistency of care and carer. Hearing from the patients themselves or reading about their histories can be very distressing. It is difficult to comprehend any one human being, especially during infancy or childhood, enduring so much suffering and pain. I am frequently amazed that the patients I have worked with survived their early lives. However, a consequence of such traumatic early lives is that their emotional and personality development has been distorted or arrested.

Each phase of human development, according to Freud (Bateman, Brown and Pedder 2000), needs to be experienced by the infant to a 'good enough' (Abram 1996) level so the infant can master the task of that phase of development before moving forward towards adulthood in their emotional and personality growth. If trauma is experienced in the pre-verbal phase of development, associated processes may not be worked through, good enough or mastered. Consequently, forensic patients who have experienced trauma in infancy often utilize pre-verbal defence mechanisms in adulthood. Those necessary defences now become pathological as there is a predominant use of them to manage emotional states during inappropriate developmental phases. Patients' internal worlds are fragmented and/or unintergrated so they use very primitive defence mechanisms such as those described by Freud as projection, repression and denial (Laplanche and Pontalis 1988), and those described by Klein as projective identification and splitting of the object (Hinshelwood 1991). It is those defences, however inappropriately they are used, that aid a patient's survival.

In the forensic setting, patients' earliest childhood experiences with their mother or primary carer are often re-enacted with nursing staff and, in a triangular sense, with their consultant psychiatrist and primary nurse. By this I mean that patients can unconsciously relate to a nurse as if they were their original mother figure. This usually means an abusive relationship dynamic. When there has been trauma in the patient's earliest life, they may not have experienced good enough psychological containment. It is this process of containment that W.R. Bion considered a necessary, fundamental process, essential for any infant to develop into an emotionally balanced, thinking adult. The process of containment is placed at the developmental stages of birth and infancy, a pre-verbal state of being, so is therefore concerned with unconscious relating initially between mother (primary carer) and infant. This process continues throughout our lifetime, but if the foundations of a good enough experience are not laid in infancy, emotional regulation in adult life becomes maladaptive.

CONTAINMENT

The concept has its origins in Melanie Klein's (1946) description of projective identification (Klein 1975). However, 1962 saw the publication of W.R. Bion's expanded works and it is he who is generally credited with coining the term 'psychological containment', as a concept in his book *Learning from Experience* (Bion 1962).

Klein (1975) described how the infant will want to get rid of unwanted parts of himself and will not want to experience his mother in a way that leaves him with negative feelings about her, as this will cause him anxiety and distress. The infant gets rid of intolerable feelings by projecting them into his mother. According to Klein, the infant does this in order to dominate and control her, take over her capacities and make them his own, and invade and destroy her. The powerful defence mechanisms of projection and projective identification afford the infant the ability of avoiding any awareness of his own feelings of separateness, dependence, admiration, feelings of envy, loss or anger and acute anxieties of fearing death through annihilation. In normal development these projections lessen as the infant learns to tolerate the ambivalent feelings of love, hate and dependence for his mother. Bion expands on Klein's concept by focusing more on the role of the mother in this process of projective identification. He describes the role of the mother in her capacity to meet her infant's needs, as well as help him manage his anxiety and distress. He proposed that, in health, from the first moment of birth the mother is in a heightened state of awareness and involvement with her infant, which Bion termed a 'mother's reverie' (Hinshelwood 1991). Bion (1962) suggests an infant needs a mother who will receive his projected feelings of distress and anxiety and think about those feelings. He described this invisible process whereby the mother makes some sense of her infant's feelings and needs in terms of 'Alpha function' (Lopez-Corvo 2003, p.26).

In order to further understand psychological containment of emotions, one can describe the concept in terms of a hungry infant. When newborn the infant is unable to understand his own bodily sensations and needs, but what he is able to do is attempt a communication of his distressing feelings to his mother about his need for food by crying, appearing to fall apart or losing visual focus. His behaviour has an effect on his mother who feels his distress. This prompts her to identify what the behaviour means. In turn she then responds, say, by feeding him. If the mother has interpreted this communication correctly, he will feel satisfied. Over many repeated experiences of the above process, the infant will eventually understand and link up the sensation of hunger to being satisfied by mother feeding him. As well as taking in food necessary for survival, the infant receives from his mother, through introjections, an experience of being understood and comforted by her, thus internalizing a containing object. After the mother has demonstrated a capacity to tolerate the infant's distress and think about the meaning of that distress, her infant will re-introject the evacuated part of his personality from his mother. Only now it does not seem as overwhelming or frightening to him, as the mother gives back her infant's feeling state in a digested, manageable form. Through repeated experience the infant has accumulated a little understanding about himself, about his body and about the experience that he is loveable and worthy of being thought about. By a 'good enough' mother providing consistently repeated experiences over time through this process, the infant introjects the mother's capacity for love and thought. This containing function of the mother appears to be a pre-requisite for an infant's mental growth, especially his capacity to think.

The infant begins to understand himself and his external world in terms of the meaning of things and begins to tolerate himself and his feelings. He is developing a capacity to contain within himself his own anxieties and develop his own internal container through having the initial experience of a mother able to contain his personality, anxieties and feelings.

However, what happens to the infant when this healthy process is replaced by hindering factors, or deprivation that prevents containment from occurring? If the mother is unable to provide love, due to being depressed for example, Bion suggests that this results in the mother being experienced as hostile to understanding. The re-introjection of the infant's frightening parts of himself will be experienced as void of meaning and therefore unsatisfying. This is then experienced by the infant as an increase in the unmanageable feelings he projected out in the first place and is now felt by him to be even more intolerable than before the evacuation. Bion referred to this as the 'nameless dread' (Lopez-Corvo 2003, p.185). Similarly, the infant may feel excessive envy or frustration at the mother's ability to do what he cannot, which results in an increase in intolerable feeling states. It is due to this lack of emotional containment along with enduring trauma that later in life the forensic patient adopts very complex, often dangerous defence mechanisms simply to survive their unbearable emotional states.

Bion's concept of containment involves an active interpersonal process between mother and infant that involves thinking, feeling, organizing and acting. This is paralleled with the experience of developing a therapeutic relationship with a patient. The creation of sound therapeutic relationships is essential in any area of mental health care. However, in forensic mental health nursing the development of a working alliance is complicated by the potential and actual risks the patient presents to others.

Applying Bion's theory to the nurse–patient relationship, the nurse is the container and the patient the contained. The patient is seeking in the nurse someone who can hold them in mind and be consistent, present and sensitive with them. Even if the patient is unable to tolerate understanding parts of him- or herself, he or she still has a need to be understood by the nurse. By this I mean that nurses manage to hold on to their counter-transference feelings, which have been projected into them by the patient, so they can think about those feelings and reflect on them with other members of staff in attempting to understand the possible unconscious communications the patient makes. In distinguishing this theory of child development to the field of forensic mental health nursing practice, one can argue that a mother can psychologically and physically contain the violent, destructive and aggressive feelings and actions that an infant projects into her. The mother may do this by holding her angry infant and soothing him, picking him up, using eye contact or a calming tone of voice and suchlike. She may identify a practical need he wants met, like feeding. However, when caring for adult forensic patients, nurses are reliant upon each other and the security measures set in place to help them psychologically and physically contain an angry and distressed adult. Secure mental health services have three very broad security measures in common:

1. Physical security in the form of outer perimeter walls, fences, cameras and locked doors.
2. Procedural security in terms of policies, procedures and the structured day.
3. Relational security in terms of staffing levels and therapeutic relationships.

The unit structure refers to the daily running of an inpatient setting, it's therapeutic milieu and 'holding environment' (Abram 1996, p.183). The nursing team's provision of a regular daily timetable of tasks, duties and activities constitutes a 'structured day'. Please see an example in Table 8.1.

PSYCHOLOGICAL CONTAINMENT WITHIN THE PRIMARY NURSE ROLE

Case example

Xena has a long personal history of sexual and physical abuse, as do several generations of her family. Her mother was aware of Xena's sexual abuse but omitted to take protective action, she being a victim of familial sexual abuse in her own childhood. As her primary nurse, Xena frequently put me in uncomfortable positions. This started in our very first meeting.

After all administrative procedures and policies had been adhered to during Xena's admission I explained that I was to be her primary nurse. We then spent some time together as part of the nursing assessment process. During the interview she sat calmly and pleasantly told me that she 'won't be here long', that 'this isn't the place for me'. When I explained some of the facts about how the ward runs on a daily basis, she said that she wouldn't be

Table 8.1: An example of a weekly ward-based activities programme

	MONDAY	*TUESDAY*	*WEDNESDAY*	*THURSDAY*	*FRIDAY*	*SATURDAY*	*SUNDAY*
08.00hrs to 09.00hrs	**Breakfast** **Medication**	**Breakfast** **Medication**	**Breakfast** **Medication**	**Breakfast** **Medication**	**Breakfast** **Medication**	**Breakfast** **Medication**	**Breakfast** **Medication**
09.30hrs to 10.30hrs	Beauty Health Group	Room Cleaning	Fresh Air and Exercise	Patients Community Meeting	Music Group	Free Time	Free Time
10.45hrs to 11.45hrs	Occupational Therapy	Current Affairs Group	Occupational Therapy	Admission Support Group	Education Session	Free Time	Free Time
12.00hrs to 14.30hrs	**Lunch** **Medication** **Room Access**	**Lunch** **Medication** **Room Access**	**Lunch** **Medication** **Room Access**	**Lunch** **Medication** **Room Access** **Canteen**	**Lunch** **Medication** **Room Access**	**Lunch** **Medication** **Room Access**	**Lunch** **Medication** **Room Access**
15.30hrs to 16.30hrs	Education Session	Arts & Crafts Projects Group	Laughter Group	Home Improvement Group	Gardening Group	Cookery Group	Free Time
17.00hrs to 18.00hrs	**Dinner** **Medication**	**Dinner** **Medication**	**Dinner** **Medication**	**Dinner** **Medication**	**Dinner** **Medication**	**Dinner** **Medication**	**Dinner** **Medication**
18.00hrs to 18.30hrs	Relaxation Group Session	Relaxation Group Session	Relaxation Group Session	Relaxation Group Session	Relaxation Group Session	Free Time	Free Time
18.30hrs to 22.00hrs	Free Time	Free Time	Film Club (Voluntary)	Free Time	Free Time	Free Time	Free Time
22.00hrs	**Medication**	**Medication**	**Medication**	**Medication**	**Medication**	**Medication**	**Medication**
23.00hrs	Bedtime	Bedtime	Bedtime	Bedtime	Bedtime at 24.00hrs	Bedtime at 24.00hrs	Bedtime

doing that, as she doesn't like being told what to do. This was conveyed in a polite, smiling, courteous and playful manner. My counter-transference during this interaction was of fury. I was thinking (but not expressing), 'You will do as you are told young lady.' I became aware of my feelings of wanting to dominate her. I discussed my emotional reaction to Xena in my supervision following this initial meeting. I was then able to meet with her the next day. When, as inevitably happened in my interaction with Xena, I was aware of feelings of domination again, I then talked to her about our initial meeting and wondered with her about her capacity to 'play games' with others. I calmly asked in a curious, non-accusatory tone of voice whether she was trying to involve me in a kind of power struggle, both yesterday and right now. I then talked to her about our new relationship in terms of beginning to experience and develop more direct communications between us, over time. She smiled broadly at me, indicating some conscious sense of having tried to goad me yesterday. We were then able to explore her fears and anxieties at being transferred to this new service. This led on to her being able to tell me about her related experiences of feeling powerless and dominated in her family life.

CONTAINMENT AND THE STRUCTURED DAY

On admission, patients can often be at their most vulnerable. Initially any patient's movement off the unit to other areas of the institution is closely assessed. Patients' movement may be initially restricted for several reasons such as:

- being a high risk to others
- being newly admitted and therefore unknown to the care team
- having an unstable mental state
- having poor motivation
- requiring enhanced engagement and observation due to increased risk of self-harm or suicide.

The daily balance between security and treatment is often very challenging for any forensic mental health professional to maintain. However, in my view, the first responsibility of any forensic mental health nurse is that of providing a safe and secure setting for patients and staff. If patients do not have this fundamental safety and their environment is chaotic and dangerous, treatment will have little impact. Subsequently increased acting out and self-preservative or sadistic violence (Glasser 1979) occurs in a patient's attempt to survive. An unsafe environment is an exact replication of many patients' earliest experiences. If this is present in hospital, there will be little possibility of learning, change or maturation taking place in a treatment setting that mirrors the environment within which the original traumas occurred.

The overall function of the 'structured day' is to help nurses create and maintain an environment where patients feel held and which is also safe to work in. Nurses can maintain a safe holding environment by appreciating the importance of boundaries that are defined and constant but are balanced with a flexibility to allow for patient and staff individuality. The clearly defined and consistent expectations of the nursing and wider clinical team in the example given in Table 8.1 are that:

- All patients are to be awake and ready to start their day by an agreed time.
- Meals are served promptly at agreed set times.
- Administration and dispensing of medication occur on time at the same time each day.
- Patients attend timetabled activities in groups.
- Patients attend half an hour of relaxation therapy marking the end of the day's planned activities and the beginning of their free time.
- A time is set to demarcate the end of the day before it is time to retire to bed.

Given the high level of structure, it is of paramount importance that the patients are encouraged to contribute to the choice of activities in order to reduce the risks of institutionalization. Through community meetings patients are supported to express their needs and choices. The nurses set and maintain the containing boundary by establishing that activities, serving lunch, dispensing medication and so on, actually happen. However, within those expectations the nursing staff, patients and wider clinical team work collaboratively to decide the chosen activities.

It may be argued that the above programme is somewhat punitive and infantilizing for an adult population. However, I believe that the patients' psychopathology has arisen, in part, from inconsistency of care often beginning in infancy. Consequently, the development of a more or less intact ego function may not have been achieved. From the perspective of Freud's structural model of the mind comprising of the id, ego and superego, this patient population have strong id impulses, desires, wishes and phantasies, combined with an often harsh superego that confronts a weak ego.

Through experiencing good enough psychological containment in infancy the ego develops the capacity to manage strong, often conflicting, impulses from the id, superego and external world. It is precisely due to enduring trauma, inconsistency of care and lack of containment in the early lives of forensic patients that it has not been possible to achieve the developmental tasks of forming a more or less intact, strong enough ego and separate identity, enabling independent living. The boundaries that a team of nurses set, both within their therapeutic relationships and the daily running of a unit, can act as an external superego for these patients against which they act out their emotional states. If the nursing and wider clinical team can maintain those agreed and defined boundaries and tolerate, in a psychologically containing way, the violence and abuse the patients will inevitably express, those patients, over time, will begin to internalize an increased sense of safety and security along with an experience that they are not solely destructive, that they can be contained, are worthy of care and are lovable.

Providing a structured day for the forensic patient aims to go some way towards providing psychological containment by providing a consistent approach and expectations in contrast to their earlier experiences of chaos. It is important that nurses are able to remain within their professional roles over time, despite patients' attempts to destroy the containment they have provided. If nurses can sustain the onslaught of destructiveness, patients may develop a growing sense of security and trust in their carers to maintain therapeutic boundaries and protect them harming themselves or others. The patients should feel that nurses can relate to them therapeutically and non-judgementally. The patients need to feel that staff can accept and tolerate the good and bad parts of their personality.

THE ADMISSION WARD

Reducing and minimizing dangerous behaviours on admission wards will enable all disciplines to be physically safe enough to assess and provide the treatments needed by each patient. In the forensic setting, an admission ward should have four major roles and functions:

- completing thorough multidisciplinary assessments
- stabilization and containment of mental health problems and risk behaviours
- provision of treatments through the secure environment, therapeutic relationships and the structured day in combination with other interventions such as medication, individual therapy and physical health care
- clear treatment pathways indicating each patient's future care.

All nursing staff should understand and accept that each patient has very different levels of prior learning, capacity and motivation for change. Psychological containment provides a useful model, especially at the initial stages of each patient's transfer to a secure mental health setting. As such, a structured day is of value, even at the stage of early admission as this is when patients are most likely to be anxious and therefore in need of high levels of containment. In attempting to provide containment for patients who are experiencing high levels of anxiety and distress, nurses should recognize and contain any feelings of frustration, anger or hopelessness when the patients refuse to engage in the specific tasks set.

The patient's level of engagement would be expected to increase when:

- medication takes effect and their mental health and mood have stabilized
- they have begun to feel psychologically secure in the fact that they are admitted to hospital and their violent, threatening or intimidating behaviour will not lead to discharge; in other words that they will not be rejected from the treatment setting
- their minds are free enough from distress to contemplate new tasks
- they choose to engage in activities in an effort to move forward
- they themselves want an increased feeling of well-being.

All nurses in the team should encourage each patient to attend off-ward activities as soon as they are assessed as safe enough to do so. Off-ward activities should take priority over the on-ward programme. This reflects a more normal lifestyle whereby people leave their homes to attend work and recreational activities. Patients are able to learn more about interpersonal relationships and have opportunities to practise containing their emotional states when meeting people other than those with whom they share a living space. In health, people are generally active, self-motivated and live within societal norms and laws. Without this opportunity for activities the patients become lethargic, isolated and at times psychologically uncontained and regressed. Having a structured active day can promote fuller, holistic assessments which incorporate each patient's strengths and abilities.

During each planned activity the nurses should be monitoring, observing, interacting and clarifying their observations of each patient's behaviours, interactions, problems, attitudes and strengths, ensuring that this information is recorded accurately in the nursing notes.

Treating antisocial, maladaptive behaviours is extremely important. Within a cognitive behavioural (CBT) model, behaviours can be modified or changed to become more socially acceptable and to reduce the risk of danger to others and themselves. Nursing staff have a major role to play in bringing about behavioural changes in patients as they are in most frequent daily contact with their patients when compared with colleagues from other disciplines. Nurses can incorporate the psychodynamic theory of containment (and other psychodynamic theories) into their practice by trying to keep in their minds an understanding of possible underlying emotional states the patients are attempting to communicate by their actions. Often what is consciously expressed is the opposite of the unconscious emotional state. For example, an aggressively spoken 'Leave me alone' can be understood as 'I'm feeling very vulnerable and fragile at the moment'.

I do not wish to underestimate the enormity of translating this theory into practice. Often patients' unconscious and conscious aggression is very frightening to experience. The temptation to yield to pressure and retreat into aggression or a sense of hopelessness is at times very strong for nurses, which is why staff time and space for reflection is so vital. But, I hope, by understanding the psychological importance of maintaining boundaries the nursing team can develop more resilience, increasing their therapeutic strength through understanding.

Table 8.2, shows some broad outcomes resulting from providing a structured day for detained patients.

THE NON-COMPLIANT PATIENT

I must stress that total compliance to rules set by the nursing team is not the aim of the structured day. In my experience, the forensic patient population do not learn or change by insistence and demands to comply. An overall aim of treatment should be to help the patients develop their self-awareness and internalize different psychic experiences from those of their traumatic early childhoods. The use of psychodynamic theory is therefore helpful for nurses, providing an understanding of possible reasons for their patients' often violent behaviours, mental health and personality problems. A dynamic function of the structured day is to provide boundaried interpersonal relationships within which patients can safely act out their emotional states. What the patients need from staff are:

- a chance to heal and grow in an environment that sustains growth by working collaboratively with patients
- constancy of time, place and boundary
- empathic responsiveness and validation of emotional states and feelings
- validation of their personal experiences
- some humour
- the presence of 'hope' and that hope being kept alive when the patient cannot do so
- continuing effort and commitment
- nurses who can admit their mistakes.

When a patient adamantly refuses to attend a scheduled activity, nursing staff should attempt to use all the therapeutic interventions and communication skills at their disposal to encourage the patient to attend. It is the containment of rule-breaking behaviour and underlying emotions that is the primary focus. Often, when a patient continues to refuse, nurses can end up feeling a range of negative emotions such as anger, frustration, victimization, being dominated and conflicted. Do I spend 30 minutes trying to get the patient to attend? If so the patients who are willing to attend may not be

Table 8.2: Some therapeutic benefits of providing a structured weekly activity programme

1. Improved engagement between staff and patients
2. Improved quality of care and service provision
3. Improved self-esteem of patients and staff
4. A sense of security and safety for patients and staff
5. Promotion of therapeutic relationships between patients and staff
6. Provide structure and meaning to the patients' day
7. Improved assessments of patients' problems and strengths
8. Opportunity to learn new skills
9. Enhance the professional development of staff by leading individual and group activities
10. Clarification of nursing roles and responsibilities
11. Improved team work and communication between staff
12. Improved supportive working atmosphere

able to, as I will need more staff to help me support the one patient who is declining. The temptation is to abandon the planned activity (and indirectly blame the refusing patient) and, in my experience, it is easier to do so but only in the short term. Consequently, it becomes essential that those patients wishing to participate in the activity should be facilitated by some of the nurses on duty. The refusing patient should be monitored or offered a space to reflect on why they were unable to make use of the care offered to them. For the duration of the activity minimal social interaction should be made with the non-compliant patient as, in a behavioural sense, this reinforces destructive behaviour by the provision of special, one-to-one time with a nurse which may, for example, be the underlying unconscious wish motivating the behaviour due to feeling jealous of other patients. Obviously, in practice, this will be determined by assessment of the patient's mental state. When the planned activity is finished, the primary nurse (or other designated nurse) can then engage with the patient who was not compliant, and further reflect upon the refusal with the patient, helping the patient to increase their self-awareness with regard to the impact of their behaviour on the larger group. The process of going back to the patient to discuss their refusal is the containing function a nurse can offer. Demonstrating that their patient's behaviour is worth the primary nurse's time and thought and a repeated willingness to try to understand their refusal in terms of the communication of an unconscious emotional state is similar to Bion's containing mother function.

CONTAINMENT AND GROUP WORK

There is much psychodynamic literature on the benefits, principles and processes of group work, which I will not review here, but I will discuss a few points in relation to the structured day. Bion proposed that the containing function a mother gives to her infant was similar to a containing function the group as a whole has for each of its members. A crucial aspect of the mother's capacity to be containing for her infant is the fact that she repeatedly meets her infant's physical and psychological needs. When each group is thought about as a container, the expected time, place, duration and breaks of each group become crucial. Nurses' attempts to strive for consistency against the patient's resistance to rules become a central focus for reflection and discussion within their teams.

On admission wards especially, the management of rule-breaking behaviours, violence and the acting out of aggressive unconscious and conscious feelings can be considered one of the primary tasks of the multiprofessional team. As containment is a lifelong process, I am equating the admission units to the patient's earliest phase of development, highlighting the need for nurses working on admission units to understand containment processes in order for even the most limited therapeutic goals to be achieved.

Case example

In my experience of implementing the structured day on an admission unit in a secure mental health setting, the value of establishing a predictable routine for patients and staff became clearer. By implementing a programme of structured activities, I witnessed a significant change in the dynamics of the ward. Prior to such activities being available, the patients were escalating in their violent verbal and physical assaults on staff. I witnessed two 'gangs' or 'factions' in constant conflict. These were the nurses and the patients. The working atmosphere was one of acute anxiety, chaos and fear of a violent experience. Becoming acutely aware of this atmosphere, on one particular day, in agreement with my colleagues, we presented the patients with a choice of two activities that would be beginning in ten minutes. It was a choice between all of us going into the garden with bats and balls or staying on the ward but moving to another area to use art materials that had not been used for years. The message, however, was clear. It was that we would all engage in the chosen activity together, as one group. After about 30 minutes of refusals, angry verbal outbursts, de-escalation, talking through and understanding a little of their protests, our collective decision was to go into the garden.

The point of my giving this account is to express my view of the changes I witnessed in the dynamics of the ward. Within a week of a daily choice of activities, I saw that the nurses were much less exposed to personal verbal attacks from patients. A lot of the aggressive, unconscious wishes were now expressed in terms of protesting and refusal to attend an activity. I feel this expression of the patients' aggression seemed much more bearable and manageable for the nursing team. After a few months, the group work and the group dynamics had largely become the container for aggression and hopelessness instead of the individual nursing team members. Anxieties, chaos and fear all significantly reduced in both patients and nurses.

The main therapeutic tasks for nurses facilitating an activities programme are to maintain the boundaries of time, duration, place, breaks and activity. Their aim in facilitating group activities and therapeutic groups is to help patients to express their emotional states and rule-breaking behaviour in a safer, more socially adaptive manner. This is done through lots of discussion and thinking (both within the individual patient and within the multidisciplinary team forums) about what prompts them when they break the rules of the ward activities programme and how they feel about this behaviour. However, we must note that patients can, through unconscious processes of projective identification and splitting, divide a team. Splitting occurs for example when two nurses experience the same patient in very different ways. Nurse A may feel sympathetic towards the patient, identifying with the victim aspects of the patient's experiences, whereas Nurse B may feel dislike and harbour a secret wish to hurt the patient, identifying with the perpetrator aspects of the patient. This type of patient has not developed the integrated capacity to both love and hate the same person. Their internal worlds are split off so they relate to and communicate with people in this unintegrated way. Because staff became aware of the possibility that such unconscious communications occur frequently with their patients and between staff groups, nurses both individually and collectively can begin to think about and contain them. Like a mother with her infant, no team will provide 100 per cent consistency. However, within the structured programme certain measures can be put in place to minimize splitting and improve consistency through the following:

- Each nurse having their own clinical supervision. As well as the nurse learning more practical skills through their own supervision, the supervisor provides a containing function for the nurse's unprocessed, emotional states when working with complex psychopathologies.
- Having regular reflective practice groups for the nursing team, in which the nurses can reflect on the patient's unconscious processes and their counter-transference feelings.
- Having regular timetabled spaces such as handover periods and clinical team meetings.
- Having regular community meetings with patients to facilitate space in the day or week to ventilate their feelings. This also provides a space for staff to feed back any issues arising in a safe, containing way and to work collaboratively in decisions affecting the unit as a whole.

CONTAINMENT FOR NURSING STAFF

When nurses are caring for and managing detained patients with severe and complex psychopathologies one of the difficulties that nurses can easily find themselves in is that of providing reactive care. Nurses can move from crisis to crisis, which leaves little space to reflect and think about what has distressed them or their patients so much. This reactive care can sometimes be understood as the nurses' defence against thinking about their patients, as the experience of doing so is unbearable at times. But processing some of those unbearable feelings can provide some insight into the patient's mind and a better understanding of their use of maladaptive non-thinking defences.

An anti-therapeutic, negative consequence of providing a structured day is that staff can easily become rigid, concrete and non-thinking about the timetable. Demanding that a patient sticks rigidly to the timetable of events can also suffocate individuality and self-expression. It can create over-compliance in a patient, which is arguably even less healthy than non-compliance, suggesting the setting in of institutionalization or of superficial change. The hope is for the patient to occupy some middle ground between these poles. A team can choose to think about aspects of a patient's unconscious communications in relation to such primative defence mechanisms as have been described earlier in the chapter and collectively hold them in mind, by which I mean hold in mind both the dangerous, perpetrator aspects of the patient and their vulnerable, victim aspects.

A crucial aspect of containment in nurse–patient relationships, whether individually or in groups, is the effect of counter-transference processes. The patient brings with them a set of expectations and ways of relating based on childhood family dynamics and the initial relationship with their mother (or primary carer). These expectations are then replicated throughout their life, especially within relationships with health professionals. Anxiety, anger, conflict and unprocessed trauma can thus be acted out and worked through in the context of the transference relationship.

The counter-transference can be thought of as the nurse's emotional reaction to the way in which the patient relates to them. Counter-transference specifically refers to the feelings aroused in the nurse. Thus in order for nurses (as well as other professionals) to maintain their own mental health, those counter-transference feelings need to be thought about and contained by others professionally skilled to do so. Reflective practice, peer supervision, individual clinical supervision, personal therapy, staff support services, clinical team meetings and handover periods, I would suggest, are all necessary forums in which staff can begin to process some of the work they do and the emotions this work inevitably invokes in them. The benefits are two-fold in that nurses are better able to maintain their mental health, reducing risk of 'burnout', and the patients' care and treatment is improved.

OVERVIEW OF SERVICES

As initially stated, I have focused much of this chapter on admission units. However, I would briefly like to put those views in the context of the wider forensic mental health service. In my view, the implementation of the structured day has different benefits for staff and patients on admission, treatment and rehabilitation wards (see Table 8.3).

Table 8.3: Primary therapeutic tasks for nurses facilitating activity groups on different types of ward within the whole impatient service

ADMISSION	TREATMENT	REHABILITATION
Good achievement of the tasks set in the groups and necessary events of the day is low priority. Priority is containment of rule-breaking behaviour, aggression and other projected emotions which can be thought about by the clinical team. Preferably all activities should be on-unit or in the ward garden area. But begin to encourage off-unit activities. When stable enough mentally, introduce off-unit activities into the daily programme. This should not be solely dependent upon compliance with the on-ward programme. More activity-based group tasks, hobbies and interests and less psychological in-depth therapy group work.	Increase in the level of therapeutic psychological group work, decreasing but not eliminating activity and hobby groups. Each patient's individual programme should be mixed with off-unit and on-unit groups and activities. Containment of unconscious processes by the therapeutic groups offered and individual therapies, as well as the structured day.	Activities set at learning life skills for the future e.g., education, paid jobs, vocational services, learning of trades and crafts. Having a job to go out to and returning to the safety of the unit, where it is more likely that anxieties will be acted out, thus mirroring the life of the general community. Promotion of internalized containing objects.

In summary, for admission units the value of the structured day is primarily in providing a safe, boundaried, non-chaotic therapeutic milieu for patients and staff in which rule breaking and violent behaviours can be thought about and managed by staff who are psychologically containing for them.

For treatment units the value of the structured day is primarily in maintaining a safe, boundaried environment in which patients can work on more in-depth psychological issues and creative positive experiences and achievements. In theory, having experienced safety, security and building therapeutic relationships, patients may have begun to internalize some of this experience. This will enable them to make better use of the individual and group therapies offered to them on these wards. The meaning of containment here will be more consistent with Bion's experiences of therapeutic work.

On rehabilitation wards the value of the structured day is primarily in maintaining a safe boundaried environment so that patients can begin to test out their experiences of and feelings about moving away from an externally created safe place to increasingly work towards self-containment. The patients' ability to cope by self-monitoring, containing and regulating their daily lives and emotional states is what nurses will be assessing. Patients will inevitably argue their readiness to leave but an awareness of unconscious processes will help confirm or refute this. This is significant and comparable to the separation and individuation phases of human development.

CONCLUSION

Bion describes a mother's reverie in the dyadic relationship between mother and infant. In applying his theory to a forensic psychiatric nurse's role, I do not mean that nurses should be expected to maintain a similar state of reverie. Likewise when he expands on his theory on the containing function a group and group processes can have, he refers to psychoanalytic treatment groups. This again is very different to the kind of therapeutic relationship a forensic mental health nurse is trained to provide. However, I believe that the theoretical and clinical principles that underpin his theory of psychological containment can be understood, adapted and applied by nurses. This extra knowledge can help nurses who care for a very complex and often high risk group of patients, by enhancing their understanding of distressing emotions and increasing their sensitivity to each patient's mental health needs and problematic behaviours, by beginning to understand how and what unconscious processes affect behaviour both in patients and staff. More than this, it helps nurses understand, think about and process some of their own powerful feelings. Beginning to help the nurse to identify and distinguish their feelings as their own and separate from those belonging to the patient has, in my experience, been very helpful.

I propose that the greatest therapeutic value of the structured day on admission wards is maintenance of consistency in time, place and duration of the schedule, which is responsive to the patients' needs. It is important that nurses give careful consideration to the emotional impact upon patients of their holidays, sickness and unexpected changes in room or appointment times. Of course, I am not suggesting that nurses should not have holidays, sick time or training, only that when these breaks in work occur, thought and discussion are given to the impact this may have on the patients with whom they have a therapeutic relationship.

Discussion of refusals, protests, violence, acting out, feelings in the nurse of hopelessness, boredom, anxiety and the like around the patient's attendance of timetabled activity is the focus of exploration with the patient. Repeatedly spending time thinking about and going over an individual patient's repeated patterns of non-compliant and inappropriate behaviours in the staff forums I have suggested in this chapter augments the primary therapeutic benefit of having a structured day. In turn it is anticipated that patients will become more consciously aware of themselves and how they relate and function in the social world.

REFERENCES AND FURTHER READING

Abram, J. (1996) *The Language of Winnicott. A Dictionary of Winnicott's Use of Words.* London: Karnac Books.

Bateman, A., Brown, D. and Pedder, J. (2000) *Introduction to Psychotherapy.* 3rd edition. London: Routledge.

Bion, W.R. (1962) *Learning from Experience.* London: Heinemann.

Glasser, M. (1979) 'Some Aspects of the Role of Aggression in the Perversions.' In Rosen, I. (ed.) *Sexual Deviations.* 2nd edition. Oxford: Oxford University Press.

Hinshelwood, R.D. (1991) *A Dictionary of Kleinian Thought.* London: Free Association Books.

Klein, M. (1975) *The Writings of Melanie Klein,* Vols 1–4. London: Hogarth Press and Institute of Psycho-Analysis.

Laplanche, J. and Pontalis, J.-B. (1988) *The Language of Psychoanalysis.* London: Karnac.

Lopez-Corvo, R.E. (2003) *The Dictionary of The Work of W. R. Bion.* London: Karnac.

Sandler, J., Holder, A., Dare, C. and Dreher, A. (1997) *Freud's Models of the Mind: An Introduction.* Psychoanalytic Monograph 1. London: Karnac.

CHAPTER 9

Nursing Dangerousness, Dangerous Nursing and the Spaces in Between: Learning to Live with Uncertainties

Christopher Scanlon and John Adlam

INTRODUCTION

One peculiar characteristic of forensic work is that the capacity of the patients to act out their violent states of mind is what has resulted in their entering into treatment, rather than any more conscious motivation for treatment or recovery. This fact of their involuntary patient status means that patients' survival is literally dependent upon, if not actively under threat from, the treatment they receive from the system of care. Disastrously this hostile dependency has, from time to time, resulted in a number of mental health workers being killed and injured by their patients and many more reports into the various ways and means in which such patients have been subjected to interpersonal and institutional mistreatment.

The focus of this chapter will be on the persistent threat to *psychic* survival faced both by nurses and patients in forensic settings, how these threats become manifest in the dynamic interplay between nurses (and others within the multidisciplinary team) and those mentally disordered offender patients who are perceived to be dangerous. Our starting point is that these threats are both real and imagined and are brought about by the enforced proximity (or the avoidance of it) between nurses and patients within forensic settings. Discussion of these issues may be timely, since it has been argued forcefully that a review of mental health policies is necessary because of the failure of statutory mental health and criminal justice services effectively to resolve the dilemma of how to manage people with personality disorder who are, or are thought to be, dangerously antisocial and have not been successfully housed within existing secure provision.

GROUPISHNESS, MEMBERSHIP AND DIS-MEMBERMENT IN SOCIETY AND IN THE MIND

In previous papers (Adlam and Scanlon 2005; Scanlon and Adlam 2008) we explored the concept of homelessness as a metaphor for the 'unhoused mind' of the personality disordered patient and the unhoused quality of teams working with such patients. We conceptualized personality disorder in terms of disturbances of 'groupishness' (Bion 1961) and we suggested that a central dynamic of forensic work is that of inclusion/exclusion in the interpersonal and social contexts. We argued that faced with the inherently antisocial and/or perverse position of unhoused and disordered patients, the individual practitioner, and the system of care as a whole, fearful of the contaminating effects of the patients' 'dangerousness', is caught between conflicting and oscillating impulses: on the one hand, to exclude the patient from services ('lock them out') or to 'help' them into treatment involving removal (dis-memberment) from mainstream society and into an enforced membership of a more appropriate grouping within the forensic system ('lock them up and lock them in'). Albert Camus (1948) explores related themes of contamination, quarantine and exile using a metaphor of the plague: 'The first thing that plague brought to our town was...undoubtedly the feeling of exile – that sensation of a void within which never left us, that irrational longing to hark back to the past or else to speed up the march of time, and those keen shafts of memory that sting like fire' (Camus 1948, p.60), and the Russia of the tsars and the Soviets used both internal and external exile as means to punish the dissident and the deviant. The forensic patient in the antisocial position faces similar sanctions, whether he is locked in or out. We shall go on later to explore the peril for the forensic nurse of exile by identification or association with these patients.

Making creative use of an epidemiological metaphor in which he describes violence as like a virulent and infectious disease, Gilligan (1996) explores the ordinary violence of societal projections into the dangerous and the dispossessed. In so doing, Gilligan (1996) makes a distinction between structural and behavioural violence, seeing the latter, the behaviours of the individual, as always taking place in the context of the former, i.e. within the formal structures and strictures of society and its expectations, from all of which they are excluded. Gilligan further suggests that as a society we have a need for there to be victims of violence, power differentials and relative deprivation in order that 'we' can have a secure sense of ourselves in relation to 'them'. The disease of ordinary violence then infects and contaminates the large groups and communities we have co-constructed and from which some people are socially dis-membered and/or unhoused. Our attention is thus drawn not simply to the unhoused and/or dangerous mind in itself but to the relationship between the unhoused and the housed: each fearing the other and in their different ways inflicting violence one upon the other, either through action or omission. Indeed Gilligan maintains that it is impossible to understand societal violence without understanding the relationship between the haves and the have-nots, the rich and the poor, or to understand dangerousness except in terms of those who experience themselves as endangered.

Thus in a profound sense the people who become defined as dangerous become psychologically unhoused and socially dis-membered in the eyes of wider society. In this uncontained state of mind they may then become *actually* homeless and *really* dangerous. They then oscillate between becoming increasingly lawless outsiders, sometimes by creating gang-like 'anti-structures' of their own, and increasingly frantic attempts to force their way into the societal groupings and structures from which they feel excluded (Rosenfeld 1971). Either way they become creatures of the twilight on the way to the darkness of the night. Set in this context it is not too difficult to understand why, in this dangerous state of mind, the unhoused, in their desire to be inside, find themselves seeking literally to 'unhouse' others through burglary, robbery or arson and to dis-member through violent assault, rape and murder.

In the latter case a paradox also obtains: because in forcing their way in so violently, they will usually find there is no longer an 'inside' that can hold them; the urge to get inside becomes even more urgent and is perpetuated as a result of this failure of this wished-for containment (Hopper 2003; James

1994). Indeed, many writers have pointed towards these patterns of relating, and the societal response to it, as being a major factor in much recidivistic offending (Norton 1996). However, in another sense this cycle of the violent invasion can often be understood as an expression of longing for a safe space that could survive the attack and contain their rage and the corresponding hope that these violent impulses can be held and contained (Winnicott 1949).

We therefore suggest that, whilst having an obvious social reality, dangerousness and homelessness, in the sense in which we are using the terms here, have to do with internal states of mind as much as the physical realities of real violence or housing problems. Indeed, one tentative link between the endangerment and the unhousedness could be that, whilst a hospital in which one is detained might afford a certain psychological as well as physical security, it is not and never can be 'a home' (Adshead 2001; Foster and Roberts 1998). Viewed from this perspective, actual and symbolic 'homelessness', like real and imagined 'dangerousness', could both be seen as both symptom and communication, a sign and a signifier, of unhoused and dis-membered states of mind.

Another problem underpinning this difficult relationship between both the 'unhoused' and those securely housed, the dangerous and the endangered, is the problem of intentionality. In forensic mental health services, even more than in other health and social care agencies, we often experience ourselves, and are experienced, as agents of social control, having to back up and reinforce the generally accepted societal view that tends to see dangerous offenders, like homeless people, as intentionally dangerous or intentionally 'homeless' or both. According to this view there is a sense in which such people are seen as *choosing* their lifestyle and are deemed to be delinquent, predatory or deviant; instead of being seen also as *vulnerable* people who have been and continue to experience themselves as being victimized and/or displaced. Because their stance is viewed as resolutely antisocial and our response is essentially in the service of 'pro-social' forces, we sometimes feel obliged to coerce or compel these 'dissidents' into a more compliant group membership and/or to put them in their 'proper place'. We exile them from our societal groupings and exclude their needs from our thoughts, in ultimately futile pursuit of a much wished-for *peaceful unconsciousness* whilst we sleep safely in our metaphorical beds, in the *alarmed* houses that we build on the other side of the ever-higher walls that we construct to protect 'us' from 'them'.

GROUPISHNESS, MEMBERSHIP AND DIS-MEMBERMENT IN THE NURSING TASK AND IN THE NURSING TEAM

The forensic dilemma can be understood as consisting in a profound anxiety within the system of care about psychic survival. In this chapter we define psychic survival as the continued capacity of the individual nurse, the team in which they work and the organization as a whole to retain a clear sense of their separateness and to think their own thoughts while remaining functional and effective, under fire, within their relationships with offender patients (Gabbard and Wilkinson 1994). We would like to suggest that whilst this anxiety is undoubtedly fuelled by the reality that sometimes patients are violent to nursing staff, our view is that there are multiple other organizational, structural and societal factors which permeate to the core of the forensic environment and contribute to the maintenance of this anxiety, whether or not any physical violence is actually enacted during treatment.

We would like to discuss a number of dimensions to this problem along a number of axes. The first of these, which we have already touched upon, is inclusion/exclusion; the second is the familiar dichotomy of care/control and the third is how to be in a relationship with the dangerous patient that does not involve identification with, or detachment from, either sadistic or masochistic positions. Dangerousness as presented in the unhousedness and psychosocial dis-memberment of the forensic patient represents a threat to the psychic survival of the nurse. In our view the immediacy of this threat lies in the *fear of contagion*; in other words, the fear that the individual nurse, the nursing team, the organization and indeed society as a whole will become *infected* with dangerousness, and so become themselves unhoused and dis-membered. Nurses are particularly vulnerable and exposed to these intense anxieties because their work inherently involves them in such physical proximity to these dangerous people. This intimate proximity is expressed through attending to their physical health needs and, at times, in controlling and restraining; and is problematic precisely because of the echoes and resonances with the forensic patients' use of their own bodies to express their distress through the physicality of their violence.

We suggest that the consequent fear of contagion can emerge in one of two ways, which are in practice overlapping and difficult to distinguish. According to one version, the danger is perceived as external: the dangerousness of the patients is forced into the nurses by means of violent acts or other forms of psychically intrusive behaviour. The alternative version is that the nurses' sense of their own dangerousness, represented by unhoused and dis-membered parts of their own minds, is brought into consciousness under pressure of the attempt to sustain therapeutic relationships with the patients. A complementary danger for the patients lies in their fear that they may become infected by the nurses' hatred, which is expressed also on behalf of society as a whole, in the form of the *controlling* wish to lock them in and/or lock them up and then *also* to punish them for their crimes. Whether the risk of contagion is felt to be from without or from within, from the nursing staff or from the patients, the problem becomes circular and tautological because in any event there is no form of quarantine that can eliminate it.

The relationship between staff and patients in an inpatient, custodial forensic unit then again brings to mind the town of Oran in Camus' *La Peste* in which, when plague breaks out, both the healthy and the contaminated find themselves together forcibly cast out, into an exile that is both internal and external, by the wider society that fears contagion: '...the people here...though they have an instinctive craving for human contact, can't bring themselves to yield to it, because of the mistrust that keeps them apart. For it's common knowledge that you can't trust your neighbour, he may pass the disease to you without your knowing it, and take advantage of a moment of inadvertence on your part to infect you' (Camus 1948, p.160). They must take their chances as they may; each fearing the rage, envy and resentment of the other. Exiled by the state, longing to turn to one another for comfort but terrified of the plague spreading by these very means, the citizen of Oran matches Bion's description of 'a group animal at war, not simply with the group, but with himself for being a group animal and with those aspects of his personality that constitute his groupishness' (Bion 1961, p.131). He also shares, with the forensic inpatient nurse and the forensic patients themselves, the experience of a hostile boundary on two fronts at once: inside the city (or ward) between the 'sick' and the 'well'; but also a boundary the experience of which is in some ways closely or even intimately shared, and that is the boundary with the outside world, public opinion, government, society. In both cases the borderlands through which this boundary runs are guarded and closely watched to ensure control of imports and exports across the frontier of the system of care.

DIS-MEMBERMENT AND RE-MEMBERING IN THE NURSING TEAM

> The best lack all conviction, while the worst
> Are filled with passionate intensity (W.B. Yeats, 'The Second Coming')

Nurses in forensic settings work at what is often referred to as the 'front line', which we understand as the intersection between nurses and patients in the physically and psychologically shared environment that is the ward. Experientially, this shared space has elusive and invisible boundaries separated by a kind of 'no-man's land' which, as a further metaphor for trench warfare, results in nurses and patients daily having to await the whistle telling them to leave the swampy cold comfort that is represented by both the nursing office and the patients' dormitory and to go 'over the top' to face the enemy. As we have written elsewhere (Adlam and Scanlon 2005; Scanlon and Adlam 2008), this dynamic is similar to the way in which teams in the homelessness sector, who also tend to identify themselves as working on the front line, experience themselves having sometimes to battle to resettle homeless people who frequently do not wish to be rehoused, at least not in the sense implied by the housing options they are offered. In both of these cases the vanguard, often nursing and/or social care staff, are asked to engage the unhoused and the dangerous with all the physical and psychological intimacies of a feared hand-to-hand combat whilst also supposedly retaining an attitude of care and concern for a potential enemy.

These face-to-face, hand-to-hand, engagements inevitably involve what Roberts (1994) has described as a *self-assigned impossible* task of attempting *carefully* to engage patients who have a very low tolerance of intimacy, are intrinsically mistrustful of such caring (Gabbard and Wilkinson 1994) and who, very understandably, often respond by making clear that such approaches are not only unwelcome but are to be negated, if not actually attacked, wherever possible and by whatever means. In their excellent review of nurses' problems in looking after 'difficult patients', Kelly and May (1982) maintain that the role of the *caring* nurse [our italic] is only viable with reference to an appreciative patient. From this perspective the nurse's sense of professional self-esteem and self-worth is frighteningly close to being experienced as in the gift of the forensic patient, who may only intend to show appreciation when they can sense collusion in the anti-social or perverse position, for example in some kind of shared excitement about physicality or other more or less subtle boundary violations.

In this situation the nurse's wish, both to be helpful and to exercise social control on behalf of society-as-a-whole, meets head-on the patient's refusal to budge. A sort of dance is set up, as the irresistible force meets the immovable object, in which the lead is constantly moving back and forth across a shifting boundary characterized by the oscillating wants and needs of the carer/controller and would-be/won't-be patient. The possibility of empathic understanding is replaced with oscillating identification or detachment, as nurses defend against the anxiety that emerges in the face of their patients' distress. If the patients continue to insist on their rights while refusing to own their responsibility for taking up such help as is offered, nursing interventions can often be more like 'revenge', 'retaliation' or, at the very least, prejudice and discrimination (Johnson and Webb 1995; Kelly and May 1982; Lewis and Appleby 1988; Main 1957; Norton and Dolan 1995; Stockwell 1974).

Forensic nurses, and the institutional settings in which they work, are under continual pressure, from both external and internal sources, to inhabit unhoused and violent states of mind. They face moment-to-moment challenges to abandon the therapeutic relationship in favour of extreme positions on the axes of inclusion versus exclusion or care versus control. For example, they might find that they are limiting themselves (and one another) to practical and administrative tasks represented by their role as custodians. Indeed, Menzies (1959) suggests that these socio-technical activities and the more hierarchical structures of nursing practice became normative *in order to protect* the nurse from the *threat* of being constantly exposed to the painfulness of extremes of human suffering: an exposure that is inherent in the role. Alternatively, under fire, nursing staff may swing towards an opposite extreme in which, no longer feeling adequately housed within themselves or within the nursing team, they intrude upon the patients, losing sight of their own professional boundaries in the process. In a seminal paper Main (1957) describes nurses' attempts to defend against these types of threats by using more primitive 'splitting' mechanisms through which certain patients are defined as difficult, bad and/or dangerous and are then vilified in a largely unconscious attempt to vent rage and hate born of feeling helplessness, particularly in the face of patients who do not seem to gratify the nurses' need to be helpful by getting better. Conversely, other patients become *constructed* as *special,* which often results in unhelpful identification and collusion, in a similarly anxious attempt by practitioners to ward off feelings of helplessness.

In these ways nursing teams and organizations working with these clients frequently experience increased personal as well as professional isolation which makes them more vulnerable to becoming controlled either through identification with, or detachment from, the antisocial projections of the clients. This in turn puts overwhelming pressure on the cohesion of the teams and organizations in which they work. The organization that was established in order to work with traumatized and dis-membered people becomes itself a traumatized, dis-membered organization as staff attempt to deal with the anxiety arising from the failed dependency within the system (Hopper 2003). Efforts to come together as a team are frustrated by those 'members' of staff who are in the moment identified with the 'unhoused' and dis-membered aspects of their patients, unable to take up meaningful membership of the team within which they work.

The more the forensic patient resists their attempts to put them 'inside', the greater becomes the pressure on the isolated nurse to move further outwards, with the concomitant risk of over-reaching and going beyond the boundary. It is in this fragmented state that the kinds of group activities that provide staff members with a sense of cohesion and personal identity are avoided or abjured or attacked (Hinshelwood 1994). Any sharing of workers' experiential knowledge of the pain and trauma of the clients, in our terms, instead of being *remembered*, reflected upon and worked through within the group, is instead effectively *dis-membered* (Adlam and Scanlon 2005; Scanlon and Adlam 2008).

Hinshelwood (1999) suggests that when patients are described as 'special' or 'difficult', these statements say much more about the state of mind of the professional during these encounters. In the case of the difficult personality disordered patient he suggests that the person's patient-hood or madness is dis-membered, leaving only the experience of a bad or disordered person. In the specific case of personality disorder within the forensic setting our suggestion is that the first casualty of this process is the capacity to re-member the patients' troubled lives and violent histories (Camus' 'keen shafts of memory that stung like fire' (p.60)). Some, relating to the lost, lonely and victimized aspects of the unhoused mind of the patients, forget or dis-member the offence and how to address the patients' criminogenic needs. Others, holding on to the complementary aspect, remember only the offence and are unable to re-member the patients' humanity and suffering.

In this way both clients and staff teams come to adopt a secretly shared primary task that could be defined as the pursuit of a state in which all knowledge of distress is denied. The staff team under pressure of this kind is intent on surviving without change and individual workers unite around a morbid terror of learning from experience: they are dominated by 'basic assumption' states of mind (Bion 1961; Hopper 2003). It is at this point that the workers turn again towards the clients, this time to push them away – or worse, to *push them around.* Indeed, such have been these concerns, from time to time, that Barker (1992) suggested that a priority concern for mental health nursing should be to protect people in care from the over-zealous direction of nurses who believe that they know what is best.

Illustration: the Blom-Cooper and Fallon reports

In the report of the committee of inquiry into complaints about the treatment of women personality disordered patients in a maximum security hospital in the UK, Judge Louis Blom-Cooper and colleagues (Department of Health 1992) found incontrovertible evidence of bullying and intimidation of women personality disordered patients. It was found that these patients were subject to systemized regimes of humiliation, excessive use of seclusion and physical assault. The inquiry also found that there was a *custodial* culture, in which security for security's sake was at the expense of therapy. Patient choice and involvement in care planning was not in evidence and patient complaints were ignored and/or routinely not upheld. In this context it was found that a staff culture of intimidation and collusion made it impossible for any member of staff to dissent, such that this culture of intimidation and collusion was 'an open secret' in the wider institution, which made the recruitment of good staff impossible. As a consequence of this report, major and swingeing changes were instituted and, to all intents and purposes, a new Women's Service and a new male Personality Disorder Service with completely new staff teams were established.

Unfortunately, in a few short years there was another inquiry into complaints about the new male Personality Disorder Service (Department of Health 1999). This time the complaints suggested that the unit was being run by the patients and in support of gross enactments of their deep psychopathologies, in such ways that the staff seemed powerless to exercise any sort of therapeutic or security regime. For example, there were serious breaches of security, including ready access to illicit drugs and alcohol. There was also evidence that some patients were operating business scams and fraudulent trading from the hospital, with the involvement and collusion of staff. There were also serious breaches of patient confidentiality, including patients' confidential medical reports being available to other patients as ammunition and for trade. Pornographic material was readily available to patients and, most worryingly, convicted paedophile patients were said to have been allowed access to child visitors of other patients for their perverse gratification. The atmosphere was one in which staff felt intimidated by the patients, felt powerless to challenge their behaviour and were fearful of patient complaints. It was suggested in the report that '... it was like giving children the keys of the sweet shop' (Department of Health 1999, p.86). To quote again from Yeats' 'The Second Coming', it was indeed as if 'mere anarchy' was 'loosed upon the world'.

DISCUSSION

Although these are controversial and perhaps extreme examples, and we are conscious of commenting on this material from a distance, it clearly illustrates some of the dynamic problems associated with individual and institutional failure to deal with this central issue of feeling at home in one's professional role when working with personality disordered patients in a forensic setting. In our view staff and patients come to position one another in an oscillation between inclusion/exclusion and care/control dimensions. On the one hand staff find themselves becoming overly controlling and seeking to dominate the social spaces belonging to the patients, whilst on the other hand our attention is drawn to them being overly appeasing in a futile attempt to be housed within the interpersonal world of the patients. The apparently socially responsible and altruistic motivation of staff has become corrupted and replaced by a tendency to dogmatism, coercion and control and/or by an abdication of their professional responsibility for setting appropriate professional boundaries.

To be clear though, we are not suggesting that these oscillations, born of complex interpersonal and organizational processes, only involve swings over long periods of time such as the ten-year period described above. These oscillations exemplify the forensic dilemma that exists from moment to moment and from day to day in all forensic settings. It is because of the ubiquitous nature of such problems that it is so intrinsic to safe practice that staff working in forensic settings should feel enabled, through supervision and supportive structures, to acknowledge to themselves and to each other this clear and present dangerousness in order that they may feel at home in their professional roles.

Hopper (2003) suggests that in incohesive social systems which use the characteristic defence of *massification*, group members make various attempts to reinforce the delusion that all share the same view of what is being said or assumed. The invitation is thus to become a colluding member of a corrupt association that looks the other way as abuses are perpetrated (Department of Health 1999). In these situations Hopper (2003) suggests that the pressure to conform and comply is immense and sanctions for what Gabbard and Wilkinson (1994) describe as thinking one's own thoughts are severe. Similarly, Volkan's socio-political concept of the 'chosen trauma' (Volkan 2002) illuminates the way in which a chosen social or organizational problem becomes unconsciously selected as a *cause célèbre*, as a defence against the pain of a more *authentic* appreciation of the patients', and the nurses', *real* pain and suffering. For example, the shared *politicized* narrative of macho posturing is 'chosen' as a defensive 'non-problem' around which 'fighters' can rally and the primary task of remembering the grief associated with the original traumas is eschewed and replaced with an expression of a *grievance* which must then be taken very seriously (Garland 1982). In this sense it could be suggested that the staff team presented in the Department of Health (1992) report might unconsciously have seen themselves as people whose job it is to cleanse, or rid, society of its undesirable element through denial of basic human rights in ways which might be akin to the 'ethnic cleansing' that has been seen on wider socio-political stages across the world. Whereas the staff team described by Department of Health (1999) might unconsciously have seen themselves as an oppressed minority, whose rights have been eroded in such a way as to diminish *their* common humanity. In both cases, proper professional responsibility has been replaced with a *grievance* and the grief inherent in both positions has been acted out rather than understood.

In this environment the most dangerous person and the most dangerous position is that of 'whistle blower' who, experienced as dissident or deviant, has to be coerced, closed down, shut up or shut out. Hopper (2003) reminds us that the adoption of this sort of incohesive organizational 'basic assumption' functioning may involve a reciprocal desire for punishment as well as for revenge on others. It is based on the compulsion to repeat traumatic experiences that have been *dis-membered* rather than *re-membered* (Adlam and Scanlon 2005, Scanlon and Adlam 2008), with the result that the original trauma, which has been forgotten, is effectively re-inflicted under cover of apparent attempts at reconciliation and reparation.

In general terms, many nurses in the mental health field tend towards a professional experience of relatively low reward and status within multidisciplinary teams. Forensic mental health nurses can feel trapped inside a Cinderella service within a Cinderella service. In our experience this sense of disempowerment and professional exclusion is often aggravated by the fact that nurses and health care assistants traditionally have been and often continue to be migrants. They come from 'somewhere else', often to escape from adverse circumstances in their places of origin, and as 'outsiders' they often feel the full force of prejudices of various kinds. This in turn make them all the more susceptible to differently problematic identifications with 'victims' and 'perpetrators' – all of which contributes, little by little, to the collective wish not to remember where and what they and others are *coming from*, and so increase the difficulties of becoming members of, as opposed to dis-membered from, a thinking team.

These observations, however, are not re-presented here to blame but rather are offered in the spirit of exploration and understanding – because perhaps nowhere are these social, organizational and interpersonal feelings about danger, dangerousness and heinous-ness found in more concentrated form than in the work of nursing staff who live and work cheek by jowl with some of the most detested in our society. We make these observations by way of a plea for greater tolerance and understanding of the difficulties of staff who work in these deeply complex and conflicted environments. This tolerance may in itself be crucially important in enabling them to do a very difficult job, one for which we might wish society would show greater gratitude in terms of professional, social and financial reward. The bottom line for us is that any discussion of the difficulties inherent in forensic work must derive from the perspective that the role of forensic mental health nurses and their colleagues involves moment-to-moment encounters with clear and present dangerousness. This is so whether or not any actual violence or threat is ever acted out upon them – or indeed whether or not they enact violence or mistreatment upon these dangerously vulnerable patients.

The truth is that it is a tough job but somebody has to do it. Staff many be attracted to this work for all sorts of personal, cultural and socio-economic reasons and some of the character traits that go with these various motivations may tend towards the better and others towards the worse. However, we would go so far as to suggest that, whatever the character traits of the staff, the power of the projective processes that we have outlined would *inevitably* tend towards polarizing staff in the ways already described. Thus our aim here is not to attempt the impossible task of eliminating apparently undesirable people or undesirable feelings from the work. Rather, it is to recognize that the dynamic processes that we have highlighted are ubiquitous and inevitable; and that, in well-managed and effectively supervised teams, nursing staff might be helped to re-member both themselves and their patients in the service of providing effective care with a consequent tendency towards a healthier and safer working environment.

SOME CONCLUDING REMARKS

In this chapter we have outlined some of the dynamic processes emerging from working with some very difficult clients in some very difficult circumstances. We have suggested that ideas of psychic 'unhousedness' and psychosocial 'dis-memberment' might be useful ways of conceptualizing the clear-and-present, moment-to-moment *dangerousness* that pervades the environment of the 'forensic setting'. This dangerousness is ubiquitous and is experienced internally and externally as problematic both within the staff and within the patients who find themselves living and/or working in these very difficult settings. Skirmishes across borders are a constant reality as individual workers, teams and patients are exposed to the relentless force of antisocial and traumatizing processes. Quarantined off inside locked wards behind high walls, there are usually few opportunities, either for nurses or for their patients, to find healthy methods to process and metabolize such violent states of mind. As we have outlined, when present, such opportunities are often avoided, by all parties to the conflict, for fear of further 'contamination' by the violence or the madness of the other. We offer these conceptualizations in the hope that an understanding of the nature of this psychological and psychosocial exile, in identification with the dissident or antisocial position of the forensic population, might be better integrated into the body of forensic nursing.

REFERENCES

Adlam, J. and Scanlon, C. (2005) 'Personality disorder and homlessness: Membership and "unhoused minds" in forensic settings.' *Group Analysis 38*, 3, 452–66. (Special Issues – Group Analysis in Forensic Settings)

Adshead, G. (2001) 'Murmurs of discontent: Treatment and treatability of personality disorder.' *Advances in Psychiatric Treatment* 7, 6, 407–14.

Barker, P. (1992) 'Psychiatric Nursing.' In Butterworth, T. and Faugier, J. (eds) *Clinical Supervision and Mentorship in Nursing.* London: Chapman Hall.

Bion, W.R. (1961) *Experiences in Groups.* London: Routledge.

Camus, A. (1948) *La Peste* (*The Plague*). London: Penguin.

Department of Health (1992) *Report of the Committee of Inquiry into Complaints about Ashworth Hospital.* London: HMSO.

Department of Health (1999) *Report of the Committee of Inquiry into the Personality Disorder Unit, Ashworth Special Hospital.* London: HMSO.

Foster, A. and Roberts, V.Z. (1998) '"Not in My Back Yard": The Psychosocial Reality of Community Care.' In Foster, A. and Roberts, V.Z. (eds) *Managing Mental Health in the Community: Chaos and Containment.* London: Routledge.

Gabbard, G.O. and Wilkinson, S.M. (1994) *Management of Counter-transference with Borderline Patients.* Washington, DC: American Psychiatric Press.

Garland, C. (1982) 'Taking the non-problem seriously.' *Group Analysis 15*, 1, 4–14.

Gilligan, J. (1996) *Violence: Reflections on our Deadliest Epidemic.* London: Jessica Kingsley Publishers.

Hinshelwood, R.D. (1994) 'Attacks on the Reflective Space: Containing Primitive Emotional States.' In Schermer, V.L. and Pines, M. (eds) *Ring of Fire: Primitive Affects and Object Relations in Group Psychotherapy.* London: Routledge.

Hinshelwood, R.D. (1999) 'The difficult patient.' *British Journal of Psychiatry 174*, 187–90.

Hopper, E. (2003) *Traumatic Experience in the Unconscious Life of Groups: The Fourth Basic Assumption: Incohesion: Aggregation/Massification or (ba) I:A/M.* London: Jessica Kingsley Publishers.

James, D.C. (1994) 'Holding and Containing in the Group and in Society.' In Brown, D. and Zinkin, L.M. (eds) *The Psyche and the Social World. Developments in Group-Analytic Theory.* London: Routledge.

Johnson, M. and Webb, C. (1995) 'Rediscovering unpopular patients: The concept of social judgement.' *Journal of Advanced Nursing 21*, 3, 466–75.

Kelly, M.P. and May, D. (1982) 'Good and bad patients: A review of the literature and a theoretical critique.' *Journal of Advanced Nursing 7*, 147–56.

Lewis, G. and Appleby, L. (1988) 'Personality disorder: The patients psychiatrists dislike.' *British Journal of Psychiatry 143*, 44–9.

Main T.F. (1957) 'The ailment.' *Journal of Medical Psychology 30*, 129–45.

Menzies, I.E.P. (1959) 'A case study in the functioning of social systems as a defence against anxiety: A report on a study of the nursing services of a general hospital.' *Human Relations 13*, 95–121. Reprinted in Menzies Lyth, I. (1988) *Coutaining Anxiety in Institutions: Selected Essays.* London: Free Association Books.

Norton, K. (1996) 'Management of difficult personality disorder patients.' *Advances in Psychiatric Treatment 2*, 202–10.

Norton, K. and Dolan, B. (1995) 'Acting out and the institutional response.' *Journal of Forensic Psychiatry 6*, 317–32.

Rosenfeld, H. (1971) 'Clinical approach to the psychoanalytic theory of the life and death instincts: An investigation into the aggressive aspects of narcissism.' *International Journal of Psychoanalysis 52*, 169–78.

Roberts, V.Z. (1994) 'The Self-assigned Impossible Tasks.' In Obholzer, A. and Roberts, V.Z. (eds) *The Unconscious at Work: Individual and Organization Stress in the Human Services.* London: Routledge.

Scanlon, C. and Adlam, J. (2008) 'Homelessness and Disorder: The Challenge of the Antisocial and the Social Response.' In Kaye, C. and Howlett, M. (eds) *Mental Health Services Today and Tomorrow: Part 1: Experiences of Providing and Receiving Care.* Oxford: Radcliffe.

Stockwell, E. (1974) *The Unpopular Patient.* London: Royal College of Nursing.

Volkan, V. (2002) 'September 11 and societal regression.' 26th Annual Foulkes' lecture. *Group Analysis 35*, 4, 456–82.

Winnicott, D.W. (1949) 'Hate in the countertransference.' *International Journal of Psychoanalysis 30*, 69–74.

Yeats, W.B. (1919) 'The Second Coming.' In Yeats, W.B. (2000) *Selected Poems.* london: Penguin.

CHAPTER 10

The 'Unthought Known': Working with Men with Personality Disorder in a High Secure Setting

Neil Gordon

INTRODUCTION

In this chapter I intend to explore the impacts upon nurses of working with personality disordered men in a high secure environment. I will begin by discussing the psycho-political nature of these environments and the ambivalent attitudes society holds towards those who are cared for in these settings. This will be followed with a brief discussion of the relationship between theory and practice. In the final part of the text I will focus on the relational world of the forensic mental health nurse illustrating through a fictitious clinical supervision narrative how this ambivalence can emerge 'in the mind' and the behaviour of those who inhabit this context.

The dialectic between punishment and treatment pervades these systems. The patients in these settings are usually perpetrators – the makers of victims (Morris 2001), they have been deemed too dangerous or unacceptable to society because of the crimes they have committed or the threat they pose (Cordess 2002). As several writers have noted (Cox 1996; Hinshelwood 1993; Morris 2001) the walls of these institutions serve to exclude those within them from the outside world in order that the painfulness of the internal culture is contained and those who offend society's sensibilities can be put away and forgotten about. It should be acknowledged, as Prins (1995, p.44) points out, 'those deemed to be *mad* and *bad* will always find themselves at the bottom of the social priority pecking order, because mentally disordered offenders, who often fail to fit neatly into societal categories, are the people nobody owns'.

For those working in day-to-day contact with this disenfranchised group it is particularly important that they create space to reflect on their own motivations and attitudes regarding their patients, to help protect themselves and those in their care from distorted and destructive unconscious interpersonal dynamics. When exploring this unique context, Bowers (2002), discusses how an informant in his study of nurses working within these environments described these institutions as 'being like another country'(p.20). Bowers suggests that this metaphor usefully illustrates how these environments represent a different world with unique values, customs and language systems. This uniqueness is further emphasized by 'the high walls, ritual security measures and searches on entry, and the profound moral implications of the residents' crimes' (p.20). Bowers believes that before an understanding of practice within these complex worlds is possible, it is necessary to understand the socio-political role they fulfil. People who have committed grave crimes and 'are considered to be an immediate danger to the public because of their dangerous, violent or criminal propensities' (Prins 1995, p.66) are, as Cordess (1996) observes, responsible for the kinds of terrors bad dreams are made of.

THE RELATIONAL WORLD OF NURSES

Having briefly outlined the social role and political nature of the high secure environment I now wish to focus on the relational world of nurses who operate in this clinical context. In doing this I will be utilizing psychodynamic conceptual frameworks supported by more recent theoretical developments, namely schema therapy, emerging from the body of work developed by Jeff Young and his colleagues (Young, Klosko and Weishar 2003). Increasingly those faced with the challenge of working with complex personality presentations are adopting more integrated approaches to therapeutic work, reflecting the fact that single models fail to address the range of pathology that is present in high secure populations. I begin this task by sharing with you my approach to utilizing theory in understanding my personal experience and making sense of what is occurring in a particular clinical context. From this starting point I intend to introduce to you three characters: a patient (Gary), a nurse (Martin) and a supervisor (Andrea), utilizing the emerging narrative between these individuals to explore the psychodynamics of the high secure hospital ward. I am using psychodynamic and schema concepts because of their *usefulness* in helping me make sense of this complex social world, but I wish to set the scene with some thoughts on the relationship between theory and practice.

THEORY AND PRACTICE

Alvin Mahrer (2004) in his most recent psychotherapy text distinguishes between what he calls *theories of truth* and *models of usefulness.* In his argument he pursues both a philosophical and clinical pathway in analysing the relationship between theory and practice. Although his text is focused on psychotherapy I believe its core message is pertinent to understanding other professional activities, including forensic mental health nursing. Within the constraints of this chapter I am unable to explore his arguments in any depth but I will paraphrase the key messages to provide a background to how I will approach the writing of this chapter. Mahrer (2004) discusses his concern that psychotherapy has become overly concerned with the truth of its theoretical perspectives and pursued a narrow epistemological path in trying to prove these truths. The consequence of this for him is an obsession with measuring the measurable and missing the essence of practice which is often difficult to objectify and capture in such a positivistic way. Alternatively he utilizes what he calls models of usefulness which he defines as ways of thinking about what we are doing to help us to achieve our goals and increase our understanding of our own and others' experiences. This conceptualization is supported by the work of Polkinghorne (1992) who outlines what he refers to as 'practitioner epistemology' in describing the way practice-based helping professionals develop and learn from their direct experiences with clients and patients.

Articulating the relationship between theory and practice is central to the aims of this book which is focused on helping mental health nurses understand their clinical experiences by offering frameworks and theories that illuminate what might be going on in a clinical encounter. I start with this point because a common response I have found when teaching mental health nurses about psychodynamic concepts is that they initially find the theories difficult to comprehend until they begin to utilize them in analysing and interpreting actual clinical experiences. It is at this point that such theories become useful as they hold a capacity for addressing emotional experience and explaining the unexplainable. I share this with the reader as I believe that many of the insights we have developed about working with difficult and challenging men who have offended against others have evolved from our reactions to and reflections upon our personal clinical experiences (Gordon 2003) and as such represent what Margison (2001) refers to as 'practice-based evidence'. I am not suggesting that this is the only type of evidence that informs our practice, rather I am emphasizing how important reflective practice is in helping us make sense of our emotional reactions in this context and how direct experience of the patient group can be used to inform our clinical approach.

INTRODUCING THE PATIENT

This notion of staying close to experience and utilizing our reactions to help us understand what is going on is a cornerstone of contemporary psychodynamic thought (Leiper and Maltby 2004), captured eloquently in the concepts of transference and counter-transference. In acknowledging this, it is essential before we begin to theorise about the high secure context that we introduce into this narrative the key players in our story to help us think about the kinds of experience and presenting issues someone working in this setting might be faced with. The 'individual patient' described below represents an amalgam of many people I work with and his complex personality issues capture the diversity of presentations the nurse in this setting encounters.

The focus of our attention is 27-year-old Gary. Like the majority of his peers, in diagnostic terms Gary meets the clinical criteria for several personality disorders, including borderline, antisocial and narcissistic. He is a difficult and challenging man who does not deal well with rules and boundaries and over the last two years since his admission has attempted to subvert the security regime and push boundaries in a range of situations. These incidents have included secreting a weapon, bullying and intimidation of vulnerable patients, threatening and one actual physical assault of nursing staff. Gary is very impulsive, has difficulties with problem solving and is quick to anger.

Before admission he was involved in a series of escalating offences beginning with burglary and assault and culminating in his index offence (his reason for admission to high secure care) with a brutal murder of a stranger in the street. In his childhood Gary was sexually and physically abused by his father and was then sexually abused by care staff in the children's home where he was placed for his own safety at the age of seven. He spent the remainder of his childhood and adolescence being moved to different homes where his challenging and violent behaviour often led to expulsion. His mother had mental health problems and suffered from alcoholism. He has one younger sister whom he was very protective of as she was also abused by his father; he lost contact with her some years ago after she was taken into care. He has been abusing drugs and alcohol since the age of 12 and has already been in prison on five separate occasions. He was admitted to the high secure setting following a hostage-taking incident in prison where he cut the face of a prison officer who he claimed had threatened and tried to intimidate him. Following this incident Gary had attempted to hang himself in his cell but was cut down while still conscious. Following a tripartheid assessment by psychology, nursing and medical staff he was transferred to a hospital environment.

Key features of the case

In summarizing the features of this case that make it representative of the personality disordered client group we work with in high secure hospitals it is worth noting:

- Gary was abused physically and sexually by people who were supposed to be caring for him and has spent much of his life in invalidating social and interpersonal environments (Linehan 1993).
- Gary's offending has been escalating for some time.
- Gary meets the diagnostic criteria for several personality disorders.
- Gary has abused drugs and alcohol from an early age.
- Gary has self-harmed and attempted suicide.
- Gary has been violent both outside and within institutional settings.

- Gary has used weapons in his attacks on others.
- Gary has problems with trust.
- Gary has problems with emotional impulsivity and anger.
- Gary has lost contact with his family.

Patients like Gary cared for within the high secure hospital environment are literally 'locked up' to receive their treatments. Many, although it is acknowledged not all, of the patients within this setting could also be described as presenting psychologically as individuals with locked-up pain (Franciosi 2001), reflecting the fact that many men who have committed serious sexual and violent offences (including murder) may themselves have been victims of physical and sexual abuse throughout their lives and experienced constant invalidation of their humanity. From the early work of Anna Freud (1936), the idea that those abused in childhood identify with and internalize the aggression of those who have victimized them, thus perpetuating this abuse, has been a popular explanation for the violent behaviour of young men like Gary. More contemporary writing (Cartwright 2002) suggests that viewing early trauma and later violence in simple cause-and-effect terms can be problematic. The original interpretation was based on the view that the traumatized individual identifies with the aggressor in order to escape and defend a vulnerable abused self that is then projected into someone else. Cartwright (2002) emphasizes rather that the nature of trauma and the total situation in which it occurred needs to be fully understood when developing a psychodynamic formulation.

TROUBLED HISTORIES

It is striking when reading case histories of patients like Gary how often their formative experiences have been characterized by torture and violence, commonly perpetrated by those who should have been caring for them and keeping them safe. The complex trauma associated with these intimate abusive experiences (Van der Kolk 1996) often becomes *locked into* or hard wired into the personality. As Brewin (2003) outlines in his review of post traumatic stress disorder (PTSD), the nature of childhood trauma, particularly abuse by parents and care-givers, can impact so profoundly on personal identity and the capacity to relate to others that the individual is consistently unable to find a sense of safety in interpersonal interactions.

One way to manage this difficulty is to dissociate from the social world and keep hidden the shame, guilt and distress associated with personal experiences of trauma, including how this personal history has contributed to a capacity to hurt and victimize others (Gilligan 2000).

As a consequence of this early trauma many of those with severe personality disorder lack a predictable sense of self, experiencing difficulties with affect regulation and impulse control leading to aggression against self and others. Patients with such traumatic histories are filled with fear about the intimacy and potentially exploitative nature of therapeutic relationships. As Van der Kolk (1996) observes, since interpersonal trauma tends to occur in situations where rules are unclear, under circumstances that are secret, where issues of responsibility are often murky, patients will be extremely sensitive to the rules, boundaries and potential dangers within therapeutic encounters. In this respect, although much of such patients' pain may be locked inside and difficult to acknowledge and work with, ironically, on the surface, their emotional dysregulation and inability to cope with even minor distress can quickly lead to self-destructive and violent behaviours. Hinshelwood (2002) describes the capacity for those who have been abused in this way to create abusive relationships with those who attempt to help them, often leading to professional retaliation in the form of condemnation or seeing the patient as unworthy of help.

RELATIONAL ENCOUNTERS

To explore this dynamic in more detail I now want to focus on relational encounters, so having presented Gary to you I now want to introduce another character to this story, a forensic mental health nurse called Martin. Martin is 30 years old and was brought up in a supportive family in the East Midlands. He has one younger sister whom he is very close to and he has worked in a high secure setting as staff nurse for four years. He has been a nurse for ten years and been very successful having recently completed a postgraduate degree programme and been promoted to a Band 6 post. He has also recently completed an in-house training course with the founder of schema therapy, Jeff Young, and co-facilitates a weekly schema therapy group. Martin is Gary's named nurse, works with Gary on a one-to-one basis once a week and is part of his care team on the ward. Another character in this narrative is Martin's supervisor Andrea, who is a clinical nurse specialist in cognitive behavioural therapy and leads the schema group that

Martin co-facilitates. Andrea has completed a clinical supervision training based on using the process model developed by Hawkins and Shohet (2000).

The care context

The ward where this interaction takes place is a 16-bedded locked environment with individual side rooms and day areas. Being a high secure setting there are regular room checks and searches of patients, and the staffing levels on the ward for each shift include four qualified staff and two nursing assistants. The ward has been disrupted of late because of staff changes and shortages and staff morale is quite low. There is concern that Gary is causing a lot of anxiety in the patient and staff group by inciting other patients and regularly exhibiting antisocial and challenging behaviour with the staff. The other 15 patients are also high risk and need constant monitoring and observation. They are becoming less tolerant of Gary and several have threatened to 'sort him out' if the staff do not stop his behaviour.

It is within this type of emotionally charged and volatile environment that the forensic nurse operates, often with noble therapeutic intentions but constrained by the day-to-day reality of needy demanding patients, limited staff resources, anti-therapeutic attitudes and ongoing interpersonal and team conflict (Melia, Moran and Mason 1998). This scenario is further complicated by the fact that several of the staff want Gary moved off the ward because they see him as the cause of the bad atmosphere and are annoyed with Martin who has been advocating for Gary and trying to encourage others to understand the psychological motivation behind his behaviour.

A PROCESS MODEL OF SUPERVISION

We enter this scene in the side room of the ward where Andrea and Martin are meeting for their fortnightly clinical supervision session. To provide some structure for the session Andrea is utilizing the Hawkins and Shohet (2000) process model of supervision which encourages the supervisee to think about the presentation of the patient (level 1), the helpers' interventions (level 2), the wider contextual factors impacting on the relationship (level 3), how the relationship is impacting on the helper (level 4) and how effectively the supervisory relationship is supporting and challenging the supervisee (levels 5 and 6). The model is underpinned by psychodynamic theory and Andrea is very sensitive to the transferential and counter-transferential dynamics that someone like Gary can invoke in his care team (Gabbard and Wilkinson 1994).

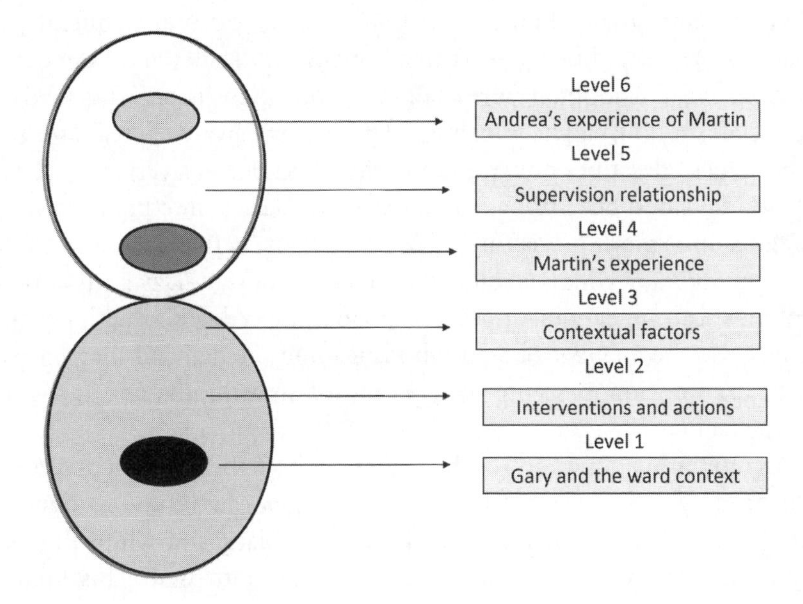

Figure 10.1: The process model of supervision

This type of process model (illustrated in Figure 10.1) is particularly useful when working with personality disorder as many of the issues that arise for nursing staff when working with this group emerge in the form of complex interpersonal dynamics which can be difficult to make sense of. The model has a systemic focus, in that it is designed to help the supervisee to connect internal world experiences with external world events and explore the inter-relationships between the personal, the relational and the contextual. A further dynamic feature of this approach is how the supervision relationship (level 5) itself becomes a focus of attention and provides a micro perspective on potential dynamics between nurse and patient that may be mirrored or paralleled in the supervision encounter.

The supervision dialogue and the Karpman Triangle

Martin informs Andrea that, when working with Gary, he finds himself being 'pulled' into being supportive and understanding as Gary discloses about his abuse and how others have treated him throughout his life. Gary is often very critical of other nursing staff whom he accuses of not caring about him and giving him a hard time, picking on him frequently for random searches and being strict in enforcing ward rules and boundaries. Gary gets very emotional when talking about these issues and tends to blame staff for how bad he is feeling. Martin is very aware of creating a split in the team so describes how he approaches this issue in a very neutral way, not taking sides but trying to understand Gary's interpretations and reactions. In exploring this further Martin discovers that the person Gary has the most issues with is an older male member of staff, Dave, who Martin recognizes can appear quite rigid and anxious in his dealings with patients. Dave is also the member of staff who is leading the demand that Gary be moved to another more secure ward because of his disruptive and uncooperative behaviour.

An interesting dimension of the scenario is how the different players are influenced by each other and how easy it is to get caught up in a dynamic where the team's thinking is split, leading to black-and-white thinking about Gary and what can and should be done with him. This kind of restricted thinking has a distinct emotional underpinning with people finding it difficult to understand and articulate their reactions to Gary. For example, Dave experiences negative feelings towards Gary and finds himself wanting to be punitive and controlling; Martin on the other hand feels compassion and empathy for Gary and is irritated with Dave and his punitive attitudes and behaviour. This is an example of what Hughes and Pengelly (1997) refer to as 'passing the painful parcel' (p.99), a reference to the Karpman Triangle which illustrates the three positions people adopt vis-à-vis one another in a conflict situation. The persecutor, the victim and the rescuer roles are often experienced at an emotional level leading to certain behaviour and interpretation of events. Dave feels like he wants to be punitive to Gary and rationalizes this behaviour as being about Gary's disruptiveness; Martin feels as if he has to rescue Gary from Dave and Gary feels that Dave is victimizing him. This is a common dynamic when working with personality disorder and needs to be explored and understood. Martin has begun to recognize this issue and taken it to his clinical supervisor to utilize this reflective space to help him make sense of his experience and deal with the challenges of the situation more effectively.

Reflecting on the goals of supervision

To reflect on the previous discussion regarding the usefulness of theory a key question at this point is: can this way of thinking about this be helpful in influencing practice and helping people deal with the complexity of this interpersonal experience? This can be tested out through the supervision process between Martin and Andrea. Andrea begins the session by creating a verbal contract asking Martin what he hopes to achieve during the encounter. Martin identifies his goals as:

- to have a greater understanding of his own feelings towards Gary and Dave
- to explore how he can handle this situation more effectively, particularly his irritation with Dave and some of the nursing team
- to explore what might be happening for Gary and why he is behaving in such a self-destructive and hostile way to other staff and patients.

Utilizing the Hawkins and Shohet (2000) model as a conversational map, Andrea began the session by asking Martin to discuss how Gary had been behaving in the ward and how staff had been responding to him. These level 1 and level 2 interventions provided the core material for the session and Martin immediately began talking about Gary feeling vulnerable and emotional, how Dave was being rigid and punitive towards him and how this was annoying him as he felt it was unprofessional. In utilizing a psychodynamic framework in understanding these perspectives it is important to think about unacknowledged unconscious feelings in all those involved (Gabbard and Wilkinson 1994).

As Hughes and Pengelly (1997) discuss in exploring the dynamic aspects of the Karpman Triangle, people will switch between the roles of persecutor, rescuer and victim often with limited awareness of what is driving their perceptions and behaviour. In psychodynamic terms the unconscious elements of this scenario can be related to transferential dynamics. It may be obvious to an external observer that Gary's problems with the autocratic and rule-enforcing Dave have distinct echoes to his relationship with his abusive father. Jeff Young *et al.* (2003) might describe this in schema terms as relating to Gary's *mistrust abuse schema*, which has developed as a consequence of his invalidating childhood environment and sexually abusive father (Gartner 1999). This schema and related emotional reactions are triggered in situations where people with authority and power are perceived to be mistreating Gary. Gary's coping response in these situations is to fight and become hostile towards his perceived abuser, acting out generally and overcompensating for his anxiety by being intimidating and rejecting towards others.

Martin, with his psychological approach to understanding this situation and his experience of Gary in the schema group, is aware of the dynamics influencing his behaviour. He therefore finds himself advocating for Gary and trying to help Dave and the rest of the team to understand what is behind his challenging behaviour. It is clear how psychological knowledge and understanding in this context can protect and help the nursing staff not to respond to Gary's behaviour as if it is directed at them personally. Dave, however, has moved to the view, highlighted by Hinshelwood (2002), that Gary is a trouble-maker and not deserving of help, encouraging his more punitive approach to dealing with him. This scenario represents the classical notion of splitting (Hughes and Pengelly 1997) where the protagonists are only able to see the situation in a polarized way. In this case, Gary is vulnerable and misunderstood or Gary is antisocial, dangerous and undeserving.

MANAGING DANGEROUSNESS AND VULNERABILITY – THE KEY TASK

This dialectical tension within the team is not about right and wrong attitudes, as someone like Gary who poses a clear risk to others needs to be viewed as both vulnerable and dangerous by those who are trying to help him. The problem to be resolved is how the staff group can be helped to hold these opposing perspectives 'in mind' and increase their understanding of what counter-transferential responses Gary is pulling out of them. Managing the capacity to maintain relational contact with a 'dangerous person' by holding on to a sense of his vulnerability and traumatic history is a central task for nurses in this setting. People like Gary can make others feel vulnerable, and have a well-developed capacity to 'put things into them'; in psychodynamic terms, projective identification. The key to managing this experience is the creation of reflective space where emotional responses can be explored, processed and understood.

Andrea encourages Martin to talk in detail about his relationship with Gary and helps him recognize his current unconscious role as rescuer; she also enables him to see how Gary is not always the victim but is also persecutory in his responses to Dave. Similarly Dave moves between the victim role as a consequence of Gary's behaviour and the persecutory role he adopts in response to Gary. Martin at times feels victimized by Dave and feels persecutory towards him in retaliation. The key issue in this scenario is how much of this is played out at an unconscious level where the three protagonists have a limited awareness of their motivations and emotional responses as they find themselves positioned in different roles.

As I highlighted at the beginning of this chapter these common dynamics are evident at all levels in the high secure context reflecting how society views those who are contained within them. By developing a framework for thinking about our emotional reactions to patients the nurse gets the chance to process feelings and explore hidden or unacknowledged aspects of the interpersonal interaction. As Bollas (1987) has discussed, often in such encounters the person registers some emotional response but finds it difficult to make sense of or articulate this experience. His delightful play on words in describing this as the 'unthought known' is particularly resonant with the experience of front-line workers who deal with dangerous and vulnerable men with personality disorder.

REFERENCES

Bollas, C. (1987) *The Shadow of the Object: Psychoanalysis of the Unthought Known.* London: Free Association Press.

Bowers, L. (2002) *Dangerous and Severe Personality Disorder: Response and Role of the Psychiatric Team.* London: Routledge.

Brewin, C.R. (2003) *Post Traumatic Stress Disorder: Malady or Myth?* New Haven, CT and London: Yale University Press.

Cartwright, D. (2002) *Psychoanalysis, Violence and Rage Type Murder: Murdering Minds.* Hove and New York: Brunner-Routledge.

Cordess, C. (1996) 'The Multidisciplinary Team: An Introduction.' In Cordess, C. and Cox, M. (eds) *Forensic Psychotherapy: Crime, Psychodynamics and the Offender Patient,* 2 vols. London: Jessica Kingsley Publishers.

Cordess, C. (2002) 'Proposals for managing dangerous people with severe personality disorder: New legislation and new follies in a new context.' *Criminal Behaviour and Mental Health 12,* 2, 12–19.

Cox, M. (1996) 'A Supervisor's View.' In Cordess, C. and Cox, M. (eds) *Forensic Psychotherapy: Crime Psychodynamics and the Offender Patient,* 2 vols. London: Jessica Kingsley Publishers.

Franciosi, P. (2001) 'The Struggle to Work with Locked-up Pain.' In Williams-Saunders, J. (ed.) *Life Within Hidden Worlds: Psychotherapy in Prisons.* London: Karnac Books.

Freud, A. (1936) *The Ego and the Mechanisms of Defence.* London: Hogarth Press.

Gabbard, G.O. and Wilkinson, S.M. (1994) *Management of Countertransference with Borderline Patients.* Northvale, NJ: Jason Aronson.

Gartner, R.B. (1999) *Betrayed as Boys. Psychodynamic Treatment of Sexually Abused Men.* New York: The Guilford Press.

Gilligan, J. (2000) *Violence: Reflections on our Deadliest Epidemic.* London: Jessica Kingsley Publishers.

Gordon, N.S. (2003) 'The swamp workers' stories: An exploration of practitioners' perspectives as a foundation for the development of a context sensitive development programme in a forensic setting.' Unpublished doctoral dissertation. Metanoia Institute/Middlesex University.

Hawkins, P. and Shohet, R. (2000) *Supervision in the Helping Professions.* Buckingham: Open University Press.

Hinshelwood, R.D. (1993) 'Locked in a role: A psychotherapist within the social defence system of a prison.' *Journal of Forensic Psychiatry 4*, 427–40.

Hinshelwood, R.D. (2002) 'Abusive help – helping abuse: The psychodynamic impact of severe personality disorder on caring institutions.' *Criminal Behaviour and Mental Health 12*, 2, 20–31.

Hughes, L. and Pengelly, P. (1997) *Staff Supervision in a Turbulent Environment: Managing Process and Task in Front-Line Services.* London: Jessica Kingsley Publishers.

Leiper, R. and Maltby, M. (2004) *The Psychodynamic Approach.* London: Sage.

Linehan, M. (1993) *Cognitive Behavioural Treatment of Borderline Personality Disorder.* New York: Guilford.

Mahrer, A.R. (2004) *Theories of Truth, Models of Usefulness.* London: Whurr Publishers.

Margison, F. (2001) 'Practice Based Evidence in Psychotherapy.' In Mace, C., Moorey, S. and Roberts, B. (eds) *Evidence in the Psychological Therapies: A Critical Guide for Practitioners.* Hove: Brunner-Routledge.

Melia, P., Moran, T. and Mason, T. (1998) 'Triumvirate nursing for personality disordered persons: Crossing the boundaries safely.' *Journal of Psychiatric and Mental Health Nursing 6*, 15–20.

Morris, M. (2001) 'Grendon Underwood: A Psychotherapeutic Prison.' In Williams Saunders, J. (ed.) *Life within Hidden Worlds. Psychotherapy in Prisons.* London: Karnac Books.

Polkinghorne, D.E. (1992) 'Postmodern Epistemology of Practice.' In Kvale, S. (ed.) *Psychology and Post Modernism.* London: Sage.

Prins, H. (1995) *Offenders, Deviants or Patients.* London: Routledge.

Van der Kolk, B.A. (1996) 'Trauma and Memory.' In Van der Kolk, B., McFarlne, A.C. and Weisaeth, L. (ed.) *Traumatic Stress. The Effects of Overwhelming Experience on Mind, Body and Society.* New York: The Guilford Press.

Young, J.E., Klosko, J.S. and Weishar, M.E. (2003) *Schema Therapy: A Practitioner's Guide.* New York: The Guilford Press.

CHAPTER 11

The Patient, her Nurse and the Therapeutic Community

Rebecca Neeld and Tom Clarke

INTRODUCTION

The therapeutic community approach is a model of care that was originally widely employed in large mental hospitals to counter the effects of institutionalization and to mobilize the residual capacity of patients suffering from chronic mental disorder for social relationships, purposeful employment and personal responsibility. There was a gradual decline in the therapeutic community movement concomitant with the decline of the large mental hospital until the 1990s when a revival of interest in therapeutic communities occurred within more specific contexts, including prisons, units for severe and borderline personality disorders, and the management of people with enduring mental illness in the community (Kennard 2000). The generalizability of the principles and practice of therapeutic community treatment to newer therapeutic communities cannot be accepted unconditionally, however, and adapted theoretical frameworks are indicated for different settings (Campling and Haigh 1999).

Therapeutic communities differ in many ways. No two are exactly alike. Each has its own personality and distinguishing features, but there are elements common to all. A therapeutic community is a total treatment system and includes psychosocial ingredients such as group activities, active client–staff interaction, client participation in decision-making and cooperation with the surrounding society (Isohanni 1993). The extent to which this takes place varies according to the setting and according to individuals' capabilities.

In general, this flattening of the traditional institutional hierarchy encourages an intimacy between patients, between the nurses and between nurses and patients. It also fosters and marshals the therapeutic elements available. In the treatment setting patients will duplicate their past traumatic histories but now, with the aid of support and insight from the whole community including nurses, fellow patients and therapists, there is the potential for beneficial change. Attention to both the symptomatic or behavioural aspects of impulsivity and the exploration of the meaning of the behaviour is used to facilitate the process of learning and change by widening the gap between conflictual mental states and impulsive action allowing more time for thinking and feeling (Masterton 1972; Norton and Dolan 1995)

In this chapter we consider the structural elements of the therapeutic community and how these serve to organize, contain and aid the therapeutic relationship. Following a brief overview of the institutional setting, we explore aspects of the therapeutic community from the patient's and then the nurse's perspective. Vignettes drawn from clinical practice are used to illuminate processes. Personal details have been changed to protect individuals' anonymity.

THE SETTING

The Cassel Hospital, near Richmond in Surrey, is a residential therapeutic community made up of three units for single adults, families and young people. The majority of patients are female and most have a diagnosis of personality disorder. Treatment may last for between two and 18 months. Patients are free to come and go and most spend weekends at their homes. Three quarters of these families, often single mothers, have been referred to the Cassel by the courts and have been assessed by social services as being unable to fulfil the needs of their children. For them, the Cassel represents a last ditch attempt to keep their families together and they run a high risk of losing custody of their children if they drop out of treatment. Although all patients enter the Cassel voluntarily, you can appreciate that these parents feel they are compelled to stay.

Treatment at the Cassel consists of a combination of psychosocial nursing and individual psychotherapy. The model of nursing care developed at the Cassel Hospital is:

- developmental – it strives towards achieving maturity be that of an individual, family, group or system
- interactionist – in that it seeks to understand complex personal, interpersonal and inter-group dynamics or collective understanding
- systemic – in terms of its objectives and methods.

(Griffiths and Leach 1998)

Each unit at the hospital has its own work and therapy groups, its own staff, nurses and psychotherapists and for part of the day, functions separately. In addition, there is a staff community team whose responsibilities cover the whole hospital. They draw up timetables for the hospital which include times for community meetings, unit meetings and work groups. They facilitate groups for new patients and for patients about to leave. They produce rotas for child-minding, for cooking and for serving meals.

The work groups are engaged upon real work essential to the institution. For the patient, contributing to the upkeep of the building or ensuring that meals are provided can help reinforce the individual's sense of value. Working with others in ordinary everyday tasks will also bring to light interpersonal problems that might otherwise remain hidden and which can then be articulated in group meetings.

The staff community team is joined by patients' representatives elected by the patients themselves to fill key positions within the hospital. Community chair persons, for example, facilitate and draw up agendas for community meetings attended by all patients four times a week. Other elected patients order provisions and organize leisure activities and housekeeping.

The object of this chapter is not to give a detailed account of the structures that the Cassel utilizes but to convey an understanding of the processes in action. However, it is important to know how the structures provide opportunities for change and understanding. A clinical vignette is presented next to illustrate this.

CASE EXAMPLE: THE PATIENT

Sarah is a 24-year-old woman and the mother of a six-year-old girl, Tessa, who is in the care of the local authority. Sarah arrived at the Cassel from prison where she was on remand awaiting trial for an offence of infanticide. A newborn baby's body had been discovered in Sarah's apartment and medical evidence showed Sarah to be the biological mother. Sarah claimed to have no knowledge of the child, of the pregnancy, the birth or death. Psychiatric expert opinion deemed that Sarah was experiencing a psychotic denial. The trial judge recommended assessment and treatment at the Cassel Hospital as an alternative to a custodial sentence.

Prior to Sarah's arrival at the Cassel a number of aspects of the case were discussed by the staff or rather a number of questions were voiced by the staff. Where in the apartment was the baby found? How long had the baby been dead? Had Sarah killed the child? Could she be around other children? Could she be safely managed at the Cassel? There were no definite answers to most of these questions but they indicate the extent of staff concerns and anxiety and implied our concerns about whether or not we could adequately nurse this woman who may have murdered a child. The staff struggled with what they already knew and with what they didn't know. This struggle was encapsulated in the staff's need to make a decision about what to tell the other patients about why Sarah was in treatment at the Cassel. To say too much too soon might run the risk of Sarah being ostracized by her fellow patients. Similarly, were the staff to appear reticent, this might arouse suspicions and the resultant fantasies could likewise result in her being ostracized.

The tension between knowing and not knowing is a constant feature of all therapeutic work and has to be made explicit and be actively managed rather than denied. The organization of the therapeutic community allows some of this to be processed and enables the creation of a potentially therapeutic space. The first step is to provide a supportive framework to enable the staff to address their anxieties, then the patients, then staff and patients together.

It was decided to tell the patients that Sarah had had two children, one who was in the care of the local authority and that the other, a baby, had died in uncertain circumstances. For the time being Sarah was only to be around children in supervised situations. Patients are used to such arrangements as many of the parents are subject to similar arrangements at least initially.

Sarah's arrival was inauspicious. She was immaculately dressed and made up, her finger nails adorned with star-spangled extensions. Sarah would speak when spoken to but would respond in monosyllables. She was reluctant to socialize and attempted to remain in her room from where she had to be fetched for groups and at meal times. She would not say anything about herself beyond that she didn't wish to be here, that she saw little sense in her being a patient. She said she would not have any more children and would have her 'tubes tied' if only the medical profession would agree to it.

Sarah was more forthcoming with the nurse who admitted her and related the circumstances that gave rise to her referral to the Cassel but in a matter-of-fact way without displaying any emotion. When Sarah spoke of her daughter, however, she was different and tears welled up in her eyes. When asked if she missed her daughter, she nodded her head slowly and deliberately. It was moments like this that made us think that despite Sarah's general presentation there was inside her shell a woman in touch with and capable of expressing her emotional life. It was this potential that led to the initial expert recommendation that she be referred to the Cassel.

Sarah's father left the family home when she was aged six. Her mother formed another relationship some years later when Sarah was aged 11 years. This man objected to Sarah's presence and she was sent to live with her father's family in Scotland. While there she was abused by a paternal cousin, a man in his late twenties. Although there had been a lack of any maternal contact, Sarah's mother asked for Sarah to return when she reached 14 years of age. Sarah acted as child-minder to her half-brothers and sisters, often missing school, while her mother went out to work. At 16 years old, Sarah left home having obtained a live-in job in a nursing home for senior citizens. She remained there for three years and left when she became pregnant by the boyfriend of the nursing home's matron. Sarah cited a family problem as her reason for leaving in order to secure references for future employment.

When she was six months pregnant Sarah returned to live with her mother and tried to find accommodation through the housing system. Following the birth of her daughter Tessa, Sarah's mother refused to have them back and they spent the next six months in bed and breakfast accommodation. Eventually Sarah and her daughter were re-housed in a hard-to-let housing estate which Sarah later described as a drug dealer's castle. One such dealer became her boyfriend. Sarah said her own drug use was minimal at this time although she did deal for her boyfriend and would often leave Tessa in his care knowing that his flat was used by addicts who would shoot up there.

Sarah then became pregnant for a second time. She received no antenatal care and avoided contact with any authorities fearing her living situation would be deemed unsuitable for bringing up children. Tessa was by this time aged three years and not yet at school. There is no record of Sarah having attended hospital to give birth. Following the discovery of the body of a baby boy in the otherwise empty flat previously occupied by Sarah, she was traced to a bed and breakfast hotel where she was staying with Tessa and where she was arrested.

The cause of death of the baby could not be ascertained. The father of the baby said that he had not been in contact with Sarah since he found out she was pregnant and did not believe the baby was his. Following Sarah's arrest, Tessa was taken into care. Whilst in prison Sarah refused to have any contact with Tessa and told her social worker that the child was better off without her and that she had never loved her daughter.

Patients bring their individual histories with them to the Cassel and the resultant ways of behaving and relating are played out against the backdrop of the hospital setting. The compulsion to repeat maladaptive behaviour patterns can be seen as a symptom of distress and be identified as such before the conclusion becomes as if 'inevitable'. With the support and insight of the whole community and the patient's individual therapist, there is the potential to differentiate between internal emotional distress and external circumstances, to understand something of the historical antecedents and the localized precipitating factors. This requires patients to strive to be as honest as possible about their past and their motivations for change. It also requires that patients and staff appreciate the loss incurred through change. For example, for some individuals the way forward involves accepting the painful fact that they are not in a position to care for their children adequately and that it is in the child's interest that the parent relinquishes their parental rights. In reaching this point most individuals will need to acknowledge the severe deprivation and abuse they suffered as children and the painful reality of the loss of their own childhood and the damage done to them.

Sarah was not obviously likeable. She showed no interest in being in the hospital and only stayed, it seemed, as an alternative to prison. In community meetings she disclosed nothing of herself and would respond with silence to direct questions or else claim she had nothing to say.

The reactions she evoked in others, both nurses and patients, were divided. Some felt very angry with her. 'What was she doing here? Why did her silence go unchallenged? Why wasn't she told that either she participates or leaves?' At times she evoked quite sado-masochistic responses and she would find herself the focus of meetings only for the participants to be frustrated by her silence. Others saw sadness in her eyes when she was asked about herself. They perceived her silences to be excruciatingly painful for her and not born of stubbornness. The discussions of our varied responses gave added understanding to Sarah's state of mind.

The only person Sarah appeared to spend time with was Jane, an adolescent girl. Jane would sometimes be enlisted by the group in a vain effort to coax Sarah into participation. Jane would generally claim not to know how Sarah was feeling or would state that she did not wish to betray her by divulging anything Sarah was not able to disclose herself. Jane did however say that Sarah often thought of her daughter and missed her. She also pointed out that Sarah was unable to remain in a room if a baby boy was present. On one occasion Sarah was observed watching toddlers at play and weeping copiously, her body motionless.

Sarah and Tessa had not met for six months and supervised contact sessions were arranged. During these sessions Sarah was stiff and awkward and she seemed unable to engage with her daughter. Following a contact session Sarah would isolate herself within her room, declining meals and refusing to speak other than to say she was 'all right' which was patently not the case. Fellow patients and staff would regularly check on her, anxious that she might harm herself.

All patients, however disturbed, are also capable of functioning in ordinary ways. By basing the life of the community on patients' work and play, the staff group are required to recognize healthy aspects of the patients, which in turn facilitates their expression (Hinshelwood 1999). Like all the other patients, Sarah was expected to participate in certain chores including cleaning and cooking. It was while cooking that she seemed much more alive and spontaneous. Sarah's suppers had been complimented and her helpfulness to the non-cooks amongst her peers was much appreciated by them. Sarah appeared to enjoy and even blossom on their positive regards. The nurse who worked alongside Sarah suggested she take on the 'job' of food ordering manager for the therapeutic community to which Sarah agreed. In this capacity, Sarah was required to attend meetings with the community staff, to work with a food ordering nurse manager and to work within an agreed budget. Sarah took the role seriously, checking menus and reminding people of expiry dates, and even reduced the existing over-spend on the food bill. She became so involved and respected that she was called upon to resolve disputes if one team used another's food allocation.

The change in Sarah's role and status heralded changes in her behaviour within community meetings. She began to offer her opinion and perceptions of others. She would remark if parents let their children run around unsupervised and on how a lack of discipline was not good for the children. When she complained that some people seemed to do as little as possible she was asked if she had ever been like that and what changed for her. She smiled at this and nodded while shrugging her shoulders. The group laughed at her predicament but in a warm and knowing way.

Sarah was by now four months into her 12-month treatment programme. There was still no mention of the dead baby in any of the community meetings. In individual sessions with her nurse and psychotherapist Sarah was able to speak of him. She acknowledged his name and that he had been named after his death when his body had been released for burial. These facts were already known. Sarah displayed no emotion in these encounters. She told her nurse that it wasn't that she didn't wish to remember; it was that she could not remember. She accepted that the boy was hers and that he was dead but she couldn't feel anything about it as she had no memory of the pregnancy or birth. Sarah's nurse reported that these communications left her feeling overwhelmingly sad and spoke about how she wanted to hold Sarah as if she were the dead baby and to give her some life. Sarah's poise and stoicism did not give vent to the expression of these emotions in a demonstrable way but the nurse did share something of these feelings with her thus bringing them closer together.

The nurse was able to use her relationship with Sarah and Sarah's trust in her to facilitate Sarah's way into the therapeutic community. The nurse ensured the other nurses were aware of Sarah's struggles, her demanding boyfriend, her schizophrenic half-sister and her uninterested callous mother. This relationship was eventually sufficiently secure and trusting enough to allow the nurse and Sarah to inform the patient group about the reasons why Sarah was not allowed to be on her own with children. The nurse told the patients that Sarah had a baby who was found dead some weeks after his birth and that the cause of death was unknown and that

Sarah had no memory of the whole thing. Sarah sat unmoving throughout, looking down at her hand with tears in her eyes.

Discussion

In the preceding vignette we can see that initially there was a space for nurses to 'discuss' the imminent referral in a way that allowed them to voice their concerns and anxieties and so be better able to think about how to best manage Sarah's introduction into the therapeutic community that would help her integrate. Sarah's inarticulateness was at times the unhelpful focus of the community meeting but alongside these were the psychosocial work groups where her talents showed through which in turn aided her self-esteem and her acceptance by her peers. This then helped her find her voice in the talking groups.

Central throughout was the role of the nurse. Sarah's key nurse participated in all aspects of Sarah's programme, and became Sarah's trusted confidante and advocate who in the context of the nurses group was able to keep a sense of hope alive in the other nurses for this woman. She was eventually able to reach a point with Sarah where together they disclosed to the community the circumstances surrounding her admission and to explain the reasons for the supervisory arrangements in place. In the following we consider in more detail the relationship between structural aspects of the therapeutic community and the role of the nurse.

CASE EXAMPLE: THE NURSE

Individual nurses are expected to act as key nurse to a small group of patients and within the context of the multidisciplinary team to agree treatment aims and care plans, to write progress nursing reports and participate in supervision with the patient's psychotherapist. Nurses commencing work within a therapeutic community setting initially feel very confused and deskilled. For one thing it can seem that the patients are more knowledgeable about how the place operates than they are. The nurse–patient relationship can be very intense with the nurse being the most readily available member of staff and thus a receptacle for the patient's projections. Managing the resultant feelings that are stirred up within the nurse is both an individual and group task. The nurse too has to strive to be honest about her feelings and to be receptive to the support and insights of her colleagues.

The most difficult situations for the nurse arise when the patient's transference relationship to her match the nurse's own experiences. In a therapeutic community setting this is inevitable. One nurse, John, complained to the nurse group that a particular patient constantly berated him for his inadequacies. The individual concerned repeatedly accused him of failing to notice her distress. She exclaimed that she would have progressed much further with a different nurse. Although John said that such complaints were voiced daily to him, another complaint was that he was never around. This particular patient had suffered abuse and neglect throughout her childhood leading to long-term fostering from the age of 11 years. She felt the foster family was all she had now and she could not complain about them or ask for more from them. Instead her pent-up fears, anxieties and frustrations were transferred onto John, her nurse. The patient, having defensively avoided the capacity to think about the mental state of others, subjects her nurse (the most available care-giver) to the hatred that she was subjected to as a child (Higgit and Fonagy 1992).

The patient's treatment of John as not 'good enough' resonated with his own personal feelings of inadequacy. He had struggled at school and was eventually diagnosed as dyslexic. His childhood peers treated him as if he were thick and he felt he was a humiliating disappointment to his parents compared to his more academically successful brother. The patient's accusations of inadequacy triggered his own feelings of inadequacy which were temporarily overwhelming and he struggled to think as well as feel.

The aim in all therapeutic endeavours is to promote thinking and feeling, followed by thoughtful, purposeful action. John had been in personal therapy himself and these painful feelings had abated to the extent that he had shared his childhood experiences with colleagues. Subsequently his colleagues were able to remind John that he had overcome his academic difficulties and that he was a valued and respected colleague whose honesty and openness were appreciated and admired. His usual capacity to think and feel was not only of value to his patients but was valued by his fellow nurses. His colleagues were thus able to help John extricate himself from fitting in with a construct of himself as inadequate. In turn this aided John in working with the patient to identify her own feelings of inadequacy arising from her multiply deprived childhood and her fear that her demands might be deemed unreasonable and lead to abandonment. Together they worked on how she could more comfortably make reasonable demands of him rather than accusing him repeatedly of failing her.

The patient in this case example found sharing particularly difficult. Unless she could have John completely to herself she would rather not have anything to do with him. This mode of behaving had cost her many relationships leaving her lonely, bitter and extremely controlling. All her disappointments were gouged out on her arms and thus a constant reminder to her that no one had ever measured up to her expectations.

According to Winnicott (1971) if a patient cannot play then something needs to be done to enable them to play, after which psychotherapy may begin. Therapy at the Cassel is supported by a psychosocial nursing action plan which is informed by our psychological understanding of the patient. As the nominated activity managers, the patient and John were required to plan a sports day together. This enabled them to play creatively, to be special, favoured even, but also to share.

Discussion

Not all nurses can bear to be this vulnerable with each other in the way John was able to be healthily dependent on his colleagues, and to seek help when it is needed. They may redouble their efforts to impress the patient, unable to acknowledge their own hatred of the patient. To conceal hate within hollow kindness, as is implied in the frequently uttered statement, 'I'm doing this for your own good,' is a particularly corrosive form of insincerity that personality disordered patients especially appear to be particularly sensitive to. At such times we must rely upon our colleagues' collective ability to be able to articulate our denied hate and anger towards the patients and to help us accept that such emotions are human and do not make us 'bad' nurses. Some nurses in John's position may become depressed or anxious, unable to call on their colleagues for support. While many nurses are able to make use of their peer group in this way and will find individual therapy helpful and enabling, others may find that this kind of work is not for them. It may be in their best interests to leave and their colleagues will be required to give them the necessary help and support to move on.

CONCLUSION

In this paper we have outlined how a therapeutic community framework can form a secure base to support both the patient and the nurse. Core elements in the therapeutic structure of the clinical setting include the time, place and purpose of different therapeutic and organizational activities, and where responsibility lies for different decisions in the service of set therapeutic goals. Staff peer support fosters knowledge of and appreciation of each other. Together with role modelling, reflective practice and supervision, peer support can create an atmosphere where nurses look out for one another and for their patients without falling into the institutional defence of locating all illness in the patients and all health in the nurses.

In a therapeutic community model of care the nurse cultivates a relationship with her patient within which feelings, thoughts and ways of relating can be talked about in as open and honest a way as possible in the here and now. The nurse is expected to use her understanding of the patient's feelings and phantasies which make him behave as he does and to use her own feelings and personal sense of self as a therapeutic medium in relation to the patient to inform therapeutic responses in varying situations (Griffiths and Leach 1998; Weddell 1968).

Creating a caring environment is a particular focus of psychiatric nursing practice (Keltner and Hogan 2003). For a proportion of patients, nurses will become the significant others in their lives, at least temporarily (Savage and McKeown 1997). Yet nurses may struggle to describe what they do in terms of an appropriate conceptual model (Mason and Chandley 1990). Therapeutic community practice is viable today, and there is currently a revival in therapeutic community products adapted to meet the needs of today's inpatient settings (Kennard 1998).

REFERENCES

Campling, P. and Haigh, R. (eds) (1999) *Therapeutic Communities: Past, Present and Future.* London: Jessica Kingsley Publishers.

Griffiths, P. and Leach, G. (1998) 'Psychosocial Nursing: A Model Learnt from Experience.' In Griffiths, P., Ord, P. and Wells, D. (eds) *Face to Face with Distress – The Professional Use of Self in Psychosocial Care.* London: Butterworth Heinemann.

Higgit, A. and Fonagy, P. (1992) 'Psychotherapy in borderline and narcissistic personality disorder.' *British Journal of Psychiatry 161*, 23–43.

Hinshelwood, R. (1999) 'Psychoanalytic Origins and Today's Work: The Cassel Heritage.' In Campling, P. and Haigh, R. (eds) *Therapeutic Communities Past, Present and Future.* London: Jessica Kingsley Publishers.

Isohanni, M. (1993) 'The therapeutic community movement in Finland: Past, current and future trends.' *Therapeutic Communities 14,* 2, 81–90.

Keltner, N.L. and Hogan, B.K. (2003) 'Introduction to Milieu Management.' In Keltner, N.L., Schwecke, L.H. and Bostrom, C.E. (eds) *Psychiatric Nursing.* St Louis, MO: Mosby.

Kennard, D. (1998) 'Editorial.' *Therapeutic Communities 19,* l, 1–2.

Kennard, D. (2000) 'Therapeutic Communities.' In Gelder, M.G., Lopez-Ibor, J.J. and Andreasen, A. (eds) *New Oxford Textbook of Psychiatry.* Oxford: Oxford University Press.

Mason, T. and Chandley, M. (1990) 'Nursing models in a special hospital: A critical analysis of efficacy.' *Journal of Advanced Nursing 15,* 667–73.

Masterton, J.F. (1972) *Treatment of the Borderline Adolescent: A Developmental Approach.* New York: Wiley.

Norotn, K. and Dolan, B. (1995) 'Acting out and institutional approaches.' *Journal of Forensic Psychiatry 6,* 2, 317–32.

Savage, L. and McKeown, M. (1997) 'Towards a new model of practice for a high dependency unit.' *Psychiatric Care 4,* 4, 182–6.

Weddell, D. (1968) 'Outline of Nurse Training – Change of Approach.' In Barnes, E. (ed.) *Psychosocial Nursing.* London: Tavistock.

Winnicott D.W. (1971) *Playing and Reality.* London: Routledge.

CHAPTER 12

Crying Out for Care

Suzanne McMillan and Anne Aiyegbusi

> But what if others cannot perceive your trauma? What if people cannot understand your desperate behaviour as the manifestation of being abused or tormented? What then? (de Zulueta 2006, p.4)

INTRODUCTION

In this chapter we will draw from our many years of clinical experience as senior nurses in a variety of secure services for women with complex mental health needs, in a range of geographical locations. The main aim of the chapter is to describe how the women patients communicate their distress through challenging behaviours and by inducing intense, negative emotional states in the nurses who are tasked with meeting their clinical needs. We will discuss how these communications can be difficult for professional care-givers to understand and respond to in therapeutic ways. The complex ways in which this population of women struggle to find care and containment will be explored. We will describe the unfortunate mental health careers that the women patients embark upon as a result of finding themselves in a system that may not have been set up to comprehend what they are trying to communicate.

We will describe how, when we worked together in a service for women in a high security psychiatric hospital, we tried to develop a nursing workforce able to intervene effectively with the complexity of care-seeking communications engaged in by women patients detained within that setting. We will describe how challenging behaviours such as self-injury and a range of interpersonal disturbances can be understood as complex care-seeking behaviours and how a nursing model based on psychodynamic practice and taking account of the patients' early trauma and attachment experiences was successfully employed to provide a therapeutic environment for women offenders with complex mental health needs and primary psychiatric diagnoses of personality disorders. We will discuss how ward-based nurses and patients in their different ways came to be understood as crying out for care in the face of overwhelming anxiety and distress associated with unprocessed traumatic phenomenology. The effect on multiprofessional relationships of working with groups of women in secure care, whose intense projections impact on everybody concerned, not just nurses, will be explored.

All the case examples in this chapter are fictitious but aim to represent the clinical material and experiences of staff and patients within secure services for women. The clinical views expressed are our own and should not be taken to reflect those of West London Mental Health NHS Trust.

WOMEN IN SECURE CARE

Of the population of women receiving secure care in the United Kingdom, most have experienced traumatic early lives with disrupted attachments and histories of abuse. Many have experienced long-term institutional care for much of their lives, often spending periods of their childhood, adolescence and adult lives in group residential settings, including closed care of one sort or another (Department of Health 2002). A frequent consequence of their negative developmental experiences is that psychologically secure, continuous and responsive care from a good enough mother or surrogate has been minimal if not apparently absent. Therefore, the capacity to reflect upon their own emotional states and those of other people has been disrupted. The ability to emotionally contain negative affect has also been severely compromised. These developmental difficulties leave the women in a serious quandary in that they are prone to externalize distress that is experienced internally while being unable to describe to others what that distress is, often leaving those who could help with the feeling of being manipulated or abused. The risk is that potentially helpful professionals actually recoil from the patients whose only known strategy is to then desperately escalate their behaviour (Gorsuch 1998, 1999).

Clinical example

Angelica is a 32-year-old woman who has a history of physical and sexual abuse within her family of origin. Both parents were violent within the home. Her mother suffered chronic depression throughout all of Angelica's childhood with frequent and lengthy hospitalizations. Sometimes Angelica remained in the family home while her mother was hospitalized. During these times she was sexually abused by her father. On other occasions Angelica was placed in the care of the local authorities and so spent periods of time in residential care. By her early teens, Angelica was regularly cutting herself and she bullied other children at school. She was eventually excluded from her comprehensive school and placed some miles away from home in a boarding school for children with special needs. While attending the boarding school she attacked another girl with a broken bottle and was subsequently remanded into custody. She spent time in a young offender institution where her self-injurious behaviour escalated and she made several suicide attempts. Angelica was transferred to a secure adolescent unit and, when she reached the age of 18, was relocated to an adult secure unit where she continued to engage in severe self-injury and other disturbed, challenging behaviours including violence to staff.

Angelica was discharged into a flat when she was 22. She led a chaotic life in the community, drinking excessively, presenting to accident and emergency departments with overdoses and making a public nuisance while there. Angelica was often involved in bar room brawls which occurred when she was intoxicated and behaved inappropriately towards other women to whom she would make disparaging remarks. In one of these brawls Angelica again assaulted a woman with a broken bottle. While on remand in prison she was assessed by a psychiatrist who felt she was depressed and in need of mental health care. As a result Angelica was admitted to a secure unit for women. While there her behaviour escalated and she engaged in severe self-injury and assaults on nurses and other patients. Angelica has remained in continuous secure psychiatric care for eight years with all attempts at rehabilitation resulting in an escalation in her disturbance. Therefore, she has remained on the intensive care ward for a considerable period of time with her care team concluding that it is unsafe to make further rehabilitation attempts. She has a primary diagnosis of borderline personality disorder.

Discussion of clinical example

In the above case example, it can be seen how Angelica was able to move through the system of childcare services through to secure psychiatric care, engaging in a range of disturbed, destructive behaviours. The links between her developmental antecedents such as history of abuse, abandonment, neglect and non-protection, and her subsequent behavioural disturbance in the form of self-injury, exclusion, insecurity, rage at her carers and assaults on others who represent her, may not be made. It is conceivable that women like Angelica who require secure mental health services due to such complex mental health needs so overwhelm the capacity of their professional carers to think about why they may behave as they do that physical containment becomes the overriding priority. However, we would suggest that in addition to physical containment, Angelica is also seeking psychological containment. Her attempts to communicate this are not heard (Hinshelwood 2002) so she escalates her attempt to communicate only to find herself further alienated from the care she seeks.

MIRRORING, NURSES AND THE MULTIPROFESSIONAL CONTEXT

The legacy of abusive care has often left women who become detained in secure settings with a propensity to re-enact traumatic experience within subsequent intimate relationships including those they have with current professional care-givers. Ward-based nurses are the professional care-givers who by virtue of their roles, most easily represent the abusive parents or other carers from the patients' pasts. As a result, nurses are particularly vulnerable to being drawn into dysfunctional interpersonal relationships among themselves, with colleagues from other disciplines and with the women patients.

In addition to the nature of nurses' roles, which involve providing continuous care based within the patients' social environments, there are other factors relating to the nursing task that leave them vulnerable to traumatic re-enactments at work. These include the intense emotional atmospheres which are usually created by the gross use of projection by patients and are often present in women's secure services. Nurses work for long periods of time in these atmospheres but are often unprepared by way of training and prior experience to understand why they feel as they do within the workplace and may have difficulty containing such extreme projections. Splitting is widespread in secure services for women and this occurs within nursing teams, frequently with polarized positions taken with regard to patients' needs and how best to meet them.

Splitting can also be pervasive within the multidisciplinary context. From the nursing perspective, feelings of being abandoned within the difficult clinical environments alone with the patients and their frightening, disturbed behaviours are commonplace, as is the feeling of struggling to cope with the patients due to being overwhelmed by intense projections and exposed to physical and emotional abuse. Most nurses working with women in secure care have been on the receiving end of extreme verbal and emotional abuse (including extreme racial abuse and harassment) and some continue to work with women who have physically assaulted them. When clinical environments cannot contain the women's psychopathology, there is a high chance that nurses will be working despite having current, physical bruising or other injuries that have been inflicted by the patients. Open emotional wounds are inevitably prevalent. This bitterly painful phenomenon puts us in mind of how some of the women patients speak about their early maltreatment and of trying to go about their childhoods full of rage and confusion with the hallmarks of battery and abuse hidden from the world, beneath their clothing. Nurses' envy about the care received by patients becomes all the more understandable. From the nurses' perspective they have been the victims of assault and abuse but it is the perpetrators of this abuse, the patients, who are offered care, concern and understanding, which in turn they appear to misuse.

When compared to nurses, colleagues from other disciplines can be experienced as being in the enviable position of having freedom to come and go as they please, avoiding patients if they sense being at risk from them. Nurses feel they have no such freedom to modulate their contact with the patients and are expected to use their own bodies in defence of their colleagues if the need arises. Senior nurses and managers are also likely to be experienced as able to skirt around the edges of ward toxicity while spending most of their working lives relatively free from negative emotionality in their offices, in interview rooms or attending meetings, for example.

A further vulnerability experienced by nurses is that they are at greater risk than are other professionals of becoming identified with their patients in the eyes of colleagues. In thinking about why this may be so, we conclude that a parallel process takes place. Infused with intolerable projections and experiencing highly disturbing affects as a result, nurses may be susceptible to attempting to seek help in ways that are in keeping with their patients' care-seeking behaviours; that is, through the professional equivalent of challenging behaviour. For example nurses who have been desperately trying to curtail a patient's relentless self-injurious behaviour and verbal abuse for hours at a time may find themselves making anger-driven remarks to senior nursing, management and clinical colleagues from other professions when an opportunity for contact occurs. Such scenarios are most likely if ward nurses feel their ordeal has not been recognized or if they feel that criticisms or further demands are being made from them.

Although unconsciously aiming to convey their feeling about what they have been exposed to, angry expressions by nurses can have the effect of creating further distance between themselves and those who may be in a position to provide support. This mirrors the patient whose desperate attempt to communicate her own struggle by impacting emotionally on nurses has in fact alienated her from the very people who are in a position to provide care and containment. Their non-ward-based colleagues may defensively avoid thinking about the nurses' presentations in terms of distress that is a manifestation of patients' projections. Of course, ward nurses themselves may not have a framework for understanding why they feel the way they do and may attribute blame onto other colleagues, hence the experience of feeling abandoned by 'management' etc. and left to work in what may be perceived as intolerable, unsafe conditions. Typically, when denied care such as supervision and emotional support from their organization, nurses tend to feel that the answer to their predicament is to increase staffing levels and may feel that 'management' is withholding resources from them.

We would argue that failure fully to think about how long periods of interpersonal work with patients impacts emotionally on nurses serves the purpose of protecting non-ward professionals from feeling guilt about the disturbance ward nurses are exposed to compared to what their working lives involve. Also, this way of practising creates distance from the feelings of impotence that are so much a part of working in the face of such severe psychopathology. Nurses are convenient receptacles for containing those difficult feelings on behalf of colleagues as well as the projections they carry for patients (Dartington 1994; Menzies Lyth 1988). For these reasons we will forcefully argue that the role of ward-based nurses in secure services for women requires detailed thought, planning and organization in a departure from traditional medical model provision. In particular, sufficient support, training, clinical leadership and supervision required for nurses to successfully undertake such emotionally exhausting work needs to be firmly in place within secure services for women before it is even possible to think about direct patient care needs.

COMPLEX CARE-SEEKING

As we have mentioned, the desperate attempt to seek care and containment is often at the heart of patients' challenging behaviours. This is paradoxical because, on the face of it, these behaviours often involve rejecting what is offered by professional care-givers, especially nurses. What we would regard as complex care-seeking includes the following difficult to manage behaviours: self-injury in all its forms, rejecting and sabotaging care plans, pressurizing nurses to operate outside of their professional roles and abusive behaviours. While we would not minimize the destructive, hateful nature of these behaviours, we would contend that there is another dimension whereby the woman patient unconsciously hopes that the professional who is emotionally impacted upon can understand how she feels, making sense of all the confusion and distress she experiences but cannot process or put into words. It is this extra dimension, we feel, that often gets overlooked by nurses who are not taught, as part of their basic training, to understand or respond to extreme complexity other than in concrete ways. For example, the patient who lies under her bedclothes with a ligature tied around her neck, shocking the nurse with whom she is developing a relationship and who discovers her, is launching an emotionally violent and sadistic attack on that nurse as well as upon herself. The patient is also trying to communicate something about the feelings she is struggling with and can only manage to do so by acting out and projecting those feelings into the nurse who finds her. It is in managing to stay on their feet and think about what this patient is communicating by reflecting on how they have been made to feel that the nurse working with women in secure care undertakes the difficult, emotional clinical work that the patient requires. In doing so the nurse can attend to the safety issues that arise from this encounter while also validating the hateful, violent and shocking feelings the patient has been struggling with and which are likely to have been stirred up by their developing therapeutic relationship.

By helping the patient to reflect upon her actions and the emotional struggles that led to them, the nurse is fulfilling a vital treatment function: that is, possibly helping the patient to develop some awareness of her out-of-control feelings and, in so doing, communicating to the patient that her 'badness' can be tolerated and that a therapeutic relationship can be sustained in the face of her insecurity. This continuation of relationship is in contrast to the rejection she had pre-empted and in some way attempted to bring about, perhaps by 'strangling' the relationship. Together, this patient and her nurse may be able to develop a care plan that takes account of the patient's difficulty in directly asking for support when she begins to feel emotionally overwhelmed.

In the years that we have worked with nurses and women patients in secure care, we have learned that the women require their front-line carers to be different from what they have had before. They want nurses to have strength, to be consistent and to have no favourites. They want to live within a contained, safe structure in which there are predictable routines. They do not want to return to the chaos they have previously known. Importantly, they want nurses to hold on to hope for them. However, through conscious and unconscious means, the women also communicate that they will test whether nurses are capable of providing all of the things they want. This is because they have learned during their early lives and thereafter that good, safe care cannot continue for long. It is this insecurity that drives the women to so often sabotage the care and relationships that nurses provide for them within the secure psychiatric setting. This insecurity manifests itself in attempts to bring about the destructive relationships and chaos with which they are so familiar but actually dread, in a pre-emptive strike before they are let down again by those tasked with their care.

For nurses, the relentless testing of their professional commitment and boundaries can feel like being battered emotionally and they can be at risk of losing their professional footing in this intensely challenging work. The patients can apply such interpersonal pressure that nurses may find themselves becoming drawn into traumatic re-enactments of devastating past relationships with carers. A patient may give the impression that she wants a collusive, dysfunctional relationship but if this is achieved, she will feel let down and her belief that this is all she will ever have will be further confirmed and reinforced. Therefore, a core task of nursing involves an important role in discontinuing the patients' maladaptive expectations of what they will get from relationships, particularly those involving people entrusted with their well-being.

THERAPEUTIC CONTAINMENT AND EMPOWERMENT

We have described above all the qualities the patients would like their nurses to possess. We are mindful of the patients' desire for idealized care-givers and how these fantasies emanate from their past deprivations. This leaves nurses at risk because they can never fulfil this idealized fantasy which in turn is experienced as provocative to the patients who have difficulty accepting less-than-ideal care (Adshead 1997). We are also aware of the psychological effects of profound dependency and the potentially debilitating consequences of long-term institutionalization. Therefore, our nursing approach emphasizes empowerment, including patients taking some responsibility for their lives as far as this is possible for offenders within a secure psychiatric setting. This empowerment can only be attempted from a solid base provided by therapeutic containment. In order to provide therapeutic containment for patients, we need first to provide a secure base (Bowlby 1988) from where nursing staff can undertake the kind of emotionally challenging clinical work we have described previously. Within our service we integrated theories of relational security and therapeutic containment into our forensic nursing practice. The main components of this model are described below.

Training

In our experience, the key to changing a nursing culture has been the provision of advanced clinical training to ward-based nurse leaders and senior nurses. A single core theoretical framework that is coherent and shared by nurses at all levels of the service and led by senior nurses at ward level has proven to be essential. In this regard we were greatly supported by the Cassel Hospital in Richmond, Surrey, where senior ward nurses were able to undertake clinical placements and advanced training in psychodynamic psychosocial nursing (see Chapter 11 in this volume for further details of the Cassel Hospital and psychodynamic psychosocial nursing). In addition to equipping nurses with the clinical skills needed to work with a challenging population of women in secure care, the provision of this training communicated to nurses that they and their work were valued and that the service was prepared to invest in them as people and as professionals. Other nurses at different levels of the organization undertook different advanced training in psychodynamic practice commensurate with their roles. All nursing staff in the service undertook short training programmes focusing on theories of attachment and psychological trauma.

A developmental perspective

A developmental perspective was applied to understanding the complex mental health needs and challenging behaviours of the women receiving care and treatment within the service. Knowledge of the patients' attachment histories and experiences of trauma also contributed to an understanding of their current relationship disturbance, negative reactions to care, risk and offending behaviours. This knowledge informed nursing interventions in the here and now and helped nurses to understand what they may have been pressurized to re-enact in their professional relationships with the patients. Knowing what role they had been cast in was key to containing rather than re-enacting a patients' traumatic history (Davies 1996).

Use of self as a therapeutic tool

The main therapeutic tool employed by nurses was their relationship with patients. Patients' care needs arising from previous attachment experiences and trauma were addressed within their relationships with nurses. Specific clinical skills applied by nurses included understanding and being responsive to conscious and unconscious communications of distress, maintaining professional boundaries in the face of pressure to transgress, self-awareness and reflectivity.

Framework for conscious and unconscious communications

Severe emotional and relationship problems arising from prior trauma and negative attachment experiences may not be accessible to patients' conscious awareness but will nevertheless be evident during interpersonal transactions with others, especially nurses and other professionals. The problems may manifest during day-to-day living in repetitive patterns of risky behaviour, physical symptoms and complex care-seeking, and the emotional impact on others. Nurses worked therapeutically with communications of distress, whether expressed consciously or unconsciously by the patients while also providing support during daily activities. Nurses took account of unconscious processes at the level of the individual, the group and the organization.

Containing structures

Prior to admission to hospital or prison, women patients' lives will usually have been in chaos. Through the physical environment of the building, systems of procedural security and the predictability of institutional routines, external containment is provided. However, containment is also required at an interpersonal level. Therapeutic activity and the opportunity to develop skills to think about rather than act out their distress took place within relationships with nurses. Examples of containing structures included community meetings and therapy programmes. Ward-based nurses provided support and worked alongside patients in these activities.

In order to provide interpersonal containment for patients, it is crucial that nurses are also provided with containing structures in the form of reflective practice and clinical supervision where they are able to process their emotional experiences at work and receive support and guidance. Ideally, group reflection and supervision should also occur within a multiprofessional context in order to prevent the kinds of projection and splitting between disciplines that we have previously described in this chapter.

Culture of enquiry

In order for nurses to provide a high level of emotional engagement with the patients, they require an environment where they can explore their practice with colleagues. This means that openness and freedom to ask questions will be expected and supported within the nursing team. A high level of emotional engagement with patients also means exposure to significant psychological disturbance of a nature that gets into professionals relationships with each other as previously described. An important component for working with this involves testing reality and, as such, a safe interpersonal environment is required. This overlaps with the need for reflective practice groups and training that discontinues the defensive ways of interacting that can be embedded in institutional settings.

Self-awareness

We have mentioned self-awareness under the sub-heading 'use of self' above. We mention it again here to emphasize how important it is for nurses to be able to reflect upon where their own vulnerabilities interact with the clinical material. This is not necessarily an easy task and it does require some skill, preferably developed within personal therapy. At the stage of working on wards, few nurses will have engaged in personal psychotherapy but some have had the opportunity to participate in experiential groups during their advanced training. Supervision and reflective practice offer opportunities to develop self-awareness skills too. The defensive practice of regarding all illness to be in patients and all health in staff was discouraged and we would take the position that like all professionals working in this field, nurses are drawn to this work in search of something for themselves that is linked to personal vulnerabilities. The sooner we all understand what that something is within ourselves, the safer and more effective we will be as practitioners. Also, we would take the view that the more we understand about our unconscious motivations, the less likely we will need to project into the patients in order to manage our lives. Our experience tells us that nurses can be vulnerable to both projecting on to, and being the recipients of projections for, other disciplines within the team so our self-awareness at work extends beyond the scope of nurses and patients to thinking about and addressing our roles within groups, teams and organizations. Ward nurses were similarly encouraged to think about themselves in relation to their work in these ways.

Empowerment

It is when therapeutic containment has been achieved that empowerment of patients to contribute more fully to their living environment can occur on a more continuous basis. We aimed for the women patients to contribute something to the care of themselves and other people. Therefore, patients were not expected to adopt the traditional sick role and nurses supported their active involvement in the service as far as each individual woman was able and within the confines of security policies and procedures. The anti-therapeutic effect of complete disempowerment was avoided. While women may be attracted to the idea of a perfect carer who can anticipate their every need in advance and respond to it, nurses were supported to understand what this fantasy was all about and how to respond to it. Nurses involved patients in the development of their care plans and in their risk assessments and plans, encouraging some ownership to be taken of their needs and some responsibility for ensuring that they were met as effectively as possible. This process of course involved nurses working with patients in terms of the way they communicated their distress. While early in the nurse–patient relationship, the nurse would accept the task of interpreting the meaning of disturbance or challenging behaviours, once this had been hypothesized, the patient was encouraged by the nurse to work towards more adaptive care-seeking. They would work in partnership towards the patient's active, ongoing management of her distress which may have involved directly requesting more input at times of increased vulnerability. The meeting of such a request was extremely important in emotionally validating women who had developed complex care-seeking behaviours as a result of repeated past invalidation.

In addition to individual needs, the ward nurses were alert to group needs and the importance of empowering the women as a community, especially at times of special vulnerability such as during the festive season. These times of increased group insecurity were addressed in the ward community meeting. It was hoped that women may raise such issues themselves but, if not, nursing staff would bring them to the ward community meeting for everyone to think about. On occasions such as the festive season, patients and nurses would acknowledge what a difficult time this was and then agree to try to work together to make it bearable at the very least and, we hoped, take the opportunity to bring the ward community together in a peaceful, caring way. All patients and nurses would then get involved in planning the holiday, producing a structured schedule of domestic and leisure activities. This kind of working together encouraged the patients to step outside of the sick role and mobilize their strengths and skills in creative ways, empowering them to make a contribution to their lives and to the ward community that could induce a sense of pride and achievement.

CONCLUSION

Women detained in secure mental health services suffering from complex mental health needs including severe personality disorders usually have two important and related strands to their phenomenology: histories of extreme childhood abuse, loss and deprivation along with current clinical presentations that include challenging behaviours which include the propensity to make other people intensely emotionally uncomfortable. These phenomena are particularly prevalent in the context of their relationships with professional carers, especially nurses. Therefore, nurses working in close interpersonal contact with the patients for long periods of time are faced with the difficult professional task of developing and maintaining therapeutic relationships with the patients. The picture is compounded by the fact that nurses are unlikely to have been equipped by their basic training to manage therapeutic relationships with patients who present with such severe psychopathology.

We found in our roles as senior nurses working in secure mental health services for women over a number of years that what is often regarded as challenging behaviour on the part of the women patients is driven by insecurity of attachment as well as traumatic re-enactment. Furthermore, while behaving interpersonally in ways that on the surface appear to reject, attack or sabotage care provided, far from aiming to drive away potential support, the women patients are actually crying out for care. What is observed behaviourally, therefore, is deceptive and detracts from the internal desperation to be understood, contained and cared for that belies their challenging behaviour. We have discussed in this chapter the parallel process that can occur with nurses when they are not able to access the training, supervision and support required to enable them to manage therapeutic relationships with such a complex population of patients. Full up with projections emanating from lengthy periods of exposure to patients who have extensive traumatic histories, nurses may communicate their need for interpersonal support through anger-driven exchanges with colleagues. We have drawn on our own experience of developing a nursing workforce within a secure mental health service for women with complex mental health needs and suggest one way to provide nurses with skills to work therapeutically within such a service. By integrating psychodynamic practice with forensic mental health nursing, we were able to provide a service whereby nurses could provide therapeutic containment for women patients who had offended and who presented with complex care-seeking behaviours.

The integration of psychodynamic practice with forensic mental health nursing involves ensuring physical and procedural safety and security while strengthening interpersonal skills. By emphasizing the interpersonal task, nurses are provided with a clear theoretical framework that takes account of unconscious as well as conscious processes. By understanding the psychological and interpersonal impact of damaged attachments, we found that nurses were able to understand patients' challenging behaviours from the perspective of anxiety and anger stirred up by the proximity of a care-giving figure. We found that applying this model enables behaviour which on the surface appears to be resistant to therapeutic interventions, to be reframed as complex care-seeking. Nurses can be helped to withstand the emotional impact of patients' intense projections by the provision of containing structures in the workplace such as psychodynamically oriented reflective practice and clinical supervision whereby they are able to process their interpersonal work in a setting where their efforts, experiences and struggles are normalized and validated.

REFERENCES

Adshead, G. (1997) '"Written on the Body": Deliberate Self Harm and Violence.' In Welldon, E.V. and Van Velsen, C. (eds) *A Practical Guide to Forensic Psychotherapy.* London: Jessica Kingsley Publishers.

Bowlby, J. (1988) *A Secure Base: Clinical Applications of Attachment Theory.* London: Routledge.

Dartington, A. (1994) 'Where Angels Fear to Tread: Idealism, Despondency and Inhibition of Thought in Hospital Nursing.' In Obholzer, A. and Roberts, V.Z. (eds) *The Unconscious at Work: Individual and Organizational Stress in the Human Services.* London: Routledge.

Davies, R. (1996) 'The Interdiscplinary Network and the Internal World of the Offender.' In Cordess, C. and Cox, M. (eds) *Forensic Psychotherapy: Crime, Psychodynamics and the Offender Patient,* Vol. II. London: Jessica Kingsley Publishers.

Department of Health (2002) *Women's Mental Health: Into the Mainstream. Strategic Development of Mental Health Care for Women.* London: HMSO.

de Zulueta, F. (2006) *From Pain to Violence: The Traumatic Roots of Destructiveness.* 2nd edition. Chichester: Whurr Publishers.

Gorsuch, N. (1998) 'Unmet need among disturbed female offenders.' *Journal of Forensic Psychiatry 9,* 3, 556–70.

Gorsuch, N. (1999) 'Disturbed female offenders: Helping the "Untreatable".' *Journal of Forensic Psychiatry 10,* 1, 98–118.

Hinshelwood, R.D. (2002) 'Abusive help – helping abuse: The psychodynamic impact of severe personality disorder on caring institutions.' *Criminal Behaviour and Mental Health 12,* 20–30.

Menzies Lyth, I. (1988) *Containing Anxiety in Institutions.* London: Free Association Books.

CHAPTER 13

Working with Suspicious Minds and Balancing Acts

Katie Downes

INTRODUCTION

The aim of this chapter is to examine some of the difficulties experienced by nurses caring for women within secure mental health services and to think about what it means to nurse, or from the perspective of the women patients, be nursed, in an environment which has to balance care and custody. The women concerned predominantly suffer from a personality disorder, some with a dual diagnosis of mental illness, and have been admitted either directly from the criminal justice system or from less secure mental health services. Furthermore, these women have experienced severe abuse, mentally, physically, emotionally and sexually and, frequently, the abuser or abusers have been their earliest significant carers. The subsequent trauma suffered by these women means that their daily living environment may inevitably become a toxic environment.

It is, therefore, important that the nursing staff have the opportunity to develop a caring strategy which incorporates an ongoing appreciation and understanding of how the women's damaged formative years have led to extremes of breakdown – mentally, socially and criminally. I have worked in secure services, with women who have a personality disorder, for over five years. During this time, both my colleagues and I have been able to access training at, for example, the Tavistock Centre and the Cassel Hospital, and had the opportunity to study psychodynamic and psychosocial nursing. These studies have enabled staff to develop understanding and knowledge about the impact of trauma and the significance of the infant's earliest relationships. Additionally, clinical experience, which linked theory and practice, has helped develop insight into the ongoing impact of the patients' relationships with their professional carers, including feelings of abandonment and rejection. Continual reflection also highlights that these feelings can be experienced by both patients and nursing staff. This in turn can lead to disturbing projections, counter-transferences and re-enactment of trauma. The intention of this chapter is, therefore, to think about such feelings and consider whether it is possible to use said feelings productively, rather than destructively or, indeed, be overwhelmed by their toxicity.

The women who are thought about in this chapter are cared for within a designated service for women but, within the organization as a whole, the majority of the patients are men, with consequential adverse effects upon the delivery of care for the women. It is important to acknowledge the government directive *Women's Mental Health: Into the Mainstream* (Department of Health 2002). This *Strategic Development of Mental Health Care for Women* highlights that there are:

> distinct differences in the social and offending profiles of women and men, their experiences of mental ill health, patterns of behaviour, their care and designed treatment needs. As women represent a small minority within a system primarily for men, their needs are poorly met. In addition women are often placed in levels of physical security greater than they need... (Department of Health 2002, p.16)

Aiyegbusi (2001) suggests the main reason for women being detained within a secure unit is their 'extreme behavioural disturbance' rather than the severity of their index offences and, furthermore, that such disturbed behaviour can be the consequence of prolonged abuse by disturbed men. It is, therefore, not difficult to argue that women need specific gender-related care, which also empowers them. Many women detained in secure services have been the victims of 'powerful' abusers such as older and stronger family members and professional carers who also possess authority within society.

These needs do not exist in a vacuum and disordered behaviour, arising from inner emotional conflict, can be experienced by both staff and patients. Thus staff disturbances can mirror patients' unconscious conflicts or, indeed, cause patient disturbances. Hughes and Pengelly (1997) discuss counter-transference and mirroring in their aptly entitled chapter 'Feelings as potential evidence' and also emphasize the importance of supervisory space in order to process and assess such evidence. In addition, they go on to address 'the gap between suspicion and evidence'. This is in relation to a child not knowing what is normal and a carer not knowing (or unable to face knowing) the reality of what is going on. As Hughes and Pengelly evocatively state, 'Both child and adult are unable to cope with love and hate towards the same person, or with confusion and uncertainty' (1997, p.93).

In the same vein, personal clinical observations indicate that nurses can have difficulties integrating opposing facets of their patients, i.e. victim/perpetrator and, furthermore, that an unconscious safe place for nursing staff to think and have emotions can reveal that they identify with one or the other facet, but rarely both. Further reflection creates the notion that patients might have difficulty integrating carer and custodian and, therefore, both patient and nurse are, arguably, equally confused and suspicious of each other. The question therefore, is: if mutually suspicious minds co-exist, could there be mutual acknowledgement of suspicion and could this acknowledgment be used as a positive force?

SUSPICIOUS MINDS WITHIN THE WARD – WHOSE ARE THEY?

From personal clinical observation and experience, it has become evident that the nursing staff work with suspicion every shift and this can mean anything from seven to 14 hours a day. As suggested earlier, this suspicion is not one-sided. The most significant suspicion may well exist within the minds of:

1. Women who have suffered severe abuse (mentally, physically and sexually) frequently inflicted by their significant carers.

And:

2. Nursing staff who care for these traumatized women within a secure environment, knowing that there may be a history of actual violence, including murder.

And equally:

3. Women who feel afraid of their carers and their carers' power.

And:

4. Nursing staff who are afraid of their patients' dangerousness.

In the Elvis Presley song *Suspicious Minds*, Elvis sings about a relationship that cannot go on with suspicious minds and how he's caught in a trap and can't walk out. The women detained within secure care cannot walk out and, no doubt, also feel 'caught in a trap'. They may well want to engage with the nurses but, from personal clinical experience, it is evident that these women are invariably suspicious and afraid of expressing themselves. Their early trauma and damaged childhood attachments have made it difficult, if not impossible, to process painful feelings through thinking and consequently, a violent physical reaction can replace thinking (Aiyegbusi 2004). This may take the form of violence to others or violent self-harm or even both. Within this toxic environment, both nurse and patient can become suspicious and afraid of the outcome of emotional exposure and both can develop defensive strategies designed to prevent the uncomfortable arousal of unresolved experiences and emotions. Thus, both parties become trapped within suspicious stalemate.

As stated earlier, the patients cannot physically walk out (although fragments of their inner worlds may have been projected elsewhere); the nurses can leave after each shift but, if fear and suspicion are not addressed, they will be taking these disturbing feelings home and both staff and patients will become, and remain, isolated and distressed. It is, therefore, inevitable that any therapeutic relationship will be adversely affected by all of 'our' suspicious minds and create and support an environment that may fuel patients to attack their care and cause staff to become caught up in painful dynamics.

ACKNOWLEDGING SUSPICIOUS MINDS

Five years of intensive personal experience of 'front-line' nursing has indicated the need to openly acknowledge the existence of suspicious minds and ultimately to mutually acknowledge their existence between nurse and patient.

Griffiths and Leach (1998) encourage the use of self as the means whereby the relationship formed between nurse and patient and the use of feelings can be developed into a productive and therapeutic communication. With this in mind, it seems imperative that we do not underestimate our suspicious minds, but rather embrace and develop them. Our feelings can guide us towards the truth and, if we can develop the ability to use our feelings productively, such feelings can become valued as a tool of enquiry and a means towards empowering patients' role in their own care.

However, there appears to be a paucity of helpful literature with regard to the use of self and the complexity of women in secure services; women, as mentioned previously, who are 'placed in levels of physical security greater than they need' (Department of Health 2002, p.16) and women whose emotional disturbance has led to their detention in secure conditions rather than the severity of their index offences. It is of no wonder that the women are suspicious and afraid, nor surprising that their nurses are equally suspicious (and arguably afraid). It seems not unreasonable to argue that projections of suspicions are abounding – the women on the whole have no reason to feel safe and secure with anyone in any position of authority and the nurses are presented with the overwhelming task of attempting to contain women with extremely unpredictable emotions and behaviour, both of which are in a constant state of flux. Clinical nursing experience eventually suggested to me that this suspicion was not something which could easily be worked through but rather something which existed and was powerful and should be acknowledged and harnessed productively. Hidden, secretive suspicion is destructive and erodes the therapeutic relationship, if not actually prohibiting the development of any engagement. By developing our feelings of suspicion (which may start off unconsciously) into open enquiry, we can help our patients do the same and provide them with a safe place where feelings can be thought about.

INTEGRATING SUSPICIOUS MINDS

But let us not underplay what an atmosphere of suspicion creates. We work in an environment of toxicity, with both our damaged and dangerous patients and our own colleagues. Due consideration of the Kleinian concept of reparation, as outlined by Hinshelwood (1989), will illustrate how a strong reparative drive can be responsible for the urge to work within one of the helping professions. Klein (1959) identified from her observations of young children that the urge to make reparation is part of growth and brings relief if guilt, or perceived guilt, is not too strong. Reparation also enriches the capacity to love. However, if persecutory anxieties are too excessive, they may impede successful personality development. These complex feelings of reparation, which may have led us to this work, evoke issues from our own pasts that are painful to address and thus the staff may simultaneously find themselves feeling raw and vulnerable, whilst caring for extremely needy patients. Our patients attack our care in many ways which can lead to staff becoming demoralized and becoming at risk of 'attacking' the patient's neediness. When patients attack our care it is invariably a communication of their distress and confusion surrounding their internal and external worlds. Our response to this communication needs to strike a balance between too little or too much control i.e. decoding what is being communicated and sharing this with our patient (and each other) so that we may attempt to empower our patient within recognizable, safe, containing boundaries, rather than disempowering by reacting unthinkingly and with measures that appear punitive and may tragically re-enact their past trauma. This is not easy and requires enormous teamwork and a culture that encourages open expressions of feelings and accessible support and supervision. In order to keep our patients (and ourselves) safe within a secure but therapeutic environment we have to develop care that is consistent and containing and this needs a thinking space. We know from experience that, where a thinking space has not been developed, our care will be attacked by colleagues as well as patients. When staff and/or patients are uncontained a culture of envy, fear and mockery can arise, with ensuing chaos.

Equally, perceived conflict between therapy and custody is further exacerbated by the nature of the secure environment. From personal and anecdotal experiences, feelings and observations, it appears that the impact of such patients can be so powerful and so toxic that the nurse may flee unthinkingly from the disturbance and, in order to alleviate the discomfort, will overcompensate with actions almost of friendship. This can result in creating a situation of care versus custody with the nurse compromising safety and security by, for example, allowing the patient a forbidden item, because the nurse perceives this as kind and helpful to the patient and, in the process, loses sight of the nature of the forensic background. Roberts (1994) describes how this denial of difference erodes the capacity for empathy and engulfs the worker in the patient's own painful despair. Ultimately this becomes an uncontained situation for both patient and staff which can result in fragmentation of both internal and external worlds.

Alternatively, the overwhelming toxic nature of the forensic background may decimate the therapeutic urge and ability of the nurse, to the extent that she can only feel safe and comfortable by addressing the perpetrator aspect of the patient and consequently acknowledge only the custodial policies of the workplace. This is also uncontaining as the victim aspect and therapeutic needs of the patients are ignored and unresolved, thus creating further splitting and fragmentation.

The uncontained chaos that results from oscillating between care and custody is difficult to dispute. Perhaps by striking a balance we can find a third position, where nurses are empowered to actually hear what patients are communicating. If we can integrate ourselves, we will gain more understanding about on how to help our patients integrate their fragmented worlds. Perhaps, also, being suspicious of our own motives as nurses will encourage a better understanding of why our patients are suspicious. Whilst a culture of enquiry is rightly valued, a culture that can also acknowledge and respect productive suspicion may well produce some robust enlightenment. Suspicion has a bad press with connotations of deceit, but it is also born out of feelings, and impressions of the existence or presence of something, and inclinations of what might or might not be believed; all of which can be bound up with projections and transferences.

CASE EXAMPLE AND DISCUSSION

The following vignette illustrates this kind of turmoil – Alice, a young woman in her early twenties, has in many ways been emotionally murdered by her mother and Alice herself attempted to physically kill her own daughter. Many years later Alice remains within a phantasy of idealizing her mother and a periodic awareness of the damage inflicted upon her by her mother. She yearns for an idealized mother but on some level is aware that her mother was far from a good enough mother. This woman has sometimes reached a point of growth where she seems free from her mother, but then the knowing of how her mother failed her and the realization and acknowledgment of her own role as a mother becomes too much. She is able to move from the paranoid-schizoid position to the depressive position for a short while but then her psychic defence is to attack or murder her care and the perversity of this defence takes the form of attacking herself, thus demonstrating to her carers how useless and valueless their care is. This is planned in such a way that the significant carer, the primary nurse (in the transference her mother) and the one to blame for her intolerable feelings, will be the one to discover her and discover her in that most extreme attack on care, attempting to kill herself.

As nurses we do struggle with integrating the victim and perpetrator aspects of patients. We also struggle with integrating the caring and custodian aspects of ourselves. Consequently, at any given time fragments of ourselves may be looking after fragments of our patients. Caring safely for all of the patient, by all of the nurse, all of the time is probably unrealistic but if we can tolerate not always achieving this, we will have reached some understanding of the attacks upon our care. To return to Alice, we identified the significant relapse signatures but, crucially, we also developed a more productive suspicious mind. For example, some time ago Alice, whilst on close observations, persuaded the nurse to give her a few seconds privacy. During those seconds Alice secreted the means to commit suicide and subsequently attempted suicide. It became evident afterwards that Alice wished to be discovered by the same nurse, and this indeed did happen. Many, many months later the scenario repeated itself and the nurse refused those seconds of privacy. When asked why by Alice, the nurse reminded her of the previous occasion. Alice accused the nurse of not trusting her and the nurse admitted that she was anxious and afraid about Alice's mental state and felt the need to be wary. Suspicion was openly acknowledged and explored and Alice given the opportunity to think about whether she was suspicious of her own mental state. Alice was empowered to have input into her own care and the opportunity to develop awareness that she was very afraid of herself and her own actions.

THERAPEUTIC REALITY ACHIEVED BY THERAPEUTIC SUSPICION

The incident described above was a reality check for patient and nurse. A time to remember and use the past. A gateway towards future engagement was opened and there was no miraculous understanding – no 'as if by magic' release from anxiety for nurse or patient – but there was an attempt by both to explore suspicion and fear. And therein lies the crux – a gateway opening is good enough, we do not need magic. When a nurse or patient is overwhelmed with horror or grief at what has happened in the past, manic defences are called in to ward off the ensuing pain and this can include denial and belittling of the offence. Consequently the task of addressing these issues is rendered so insignificant that it is 'as if it can be accomplished by magic' (Hinshelwood 1989, p.346).

If both patient and nurse can develop the ability and courage to express their suspicions, a space may then be created that is safe enough to acknowledge both the existence of disturbed thoughts and the reality of disturbed actions. Additionally, this space may be used to therapeutically voice that the issues are significant and deserve significant care, thought and work by both patient and nurse.

A BALANCING ACT

We are frequently split off into different aspects of ourselves – carer, patient, nurse, gaoler, victim, perpetrator; powerful and vulnerable. As nurses we may wish to seek refuge in only one part of the whole and can then fragment ourselves, our care, the patient and the whole team. In fact, the community of the whole unit can be torn apart. If we hope to empower our patients, we have to empower ourselves as nurses.

It is important that we look to our own vulnerability. Our patients have great fear of their vulnerability, especially after addressing issues in therapy, and this can lead to patients attacking nurses' care. There is a subsequent fear of truth, but also a fear of being lied to. There is a threat of reality. But staff too may be scared of the truth, the truth of what their patients have experienced, the truth of what their patients have done and, ultimately, the truth of how they feel about their patients. What feelings do the patients evoke in the staff? How difficult is it to be honest and how often do staff use collusion as a defence against pain, fear and an unwillingness to address the truth? Not only do patients attack care, so too do staff. There are times when we are all dishonest with our feelings. This is a toxic, painful environment and for those who live with it, that is, patients and nurses, there are times when it becomes intolerable. This is when achieving a balance is most important.

SUSPICION OF SELF AND A CASE EXAMPLE

Part of getting this balance right is to be suspicious of ourselves and develop self-awareness of our own collusion with our patients' denial as a form of defence. We are justifiably cautious of significant anniversaries in our patients' lives. But it is possible to become unbalanced about this. A chilling example concerns a middle-aged woman who, on the anniversary of her index offence, expressed her expectations of how her special day would be conducted. It became apparent that she had anticipations of being seen as if she was a 'birthday girl'. The woman's distress was validated: on this date she had been very ill and her life had changed forever, but it was also the date when she had killed her brother. We need to keep our patients safe, but somehow, in this instance, the juggling act of balancing therapy and reality had caused all the balls to fall down on one side. It would appear that we could only nurse the victim as we were too scared to nurse the perpetrator, and possibly too scared to nurse the likely overwhelming fragmentation.

BEING DISBELIEVED

Many people initially think of an attack as being physical, but in our type of work we are well aware of the traumatic effect of emotional attack upon both staff and patients. Our patients can be devastated if we do not believe them. At the same time they sometimes need to be challenged and contained. But also they need to challenge us, as their traumatic pasts have caused them to be understandably suspicious of their carers. Staff equally need to be vigilant for the safety of all patients and all staff. There is an evident need to use suspicion as a culture of enquiry and to allow both staff and patients to be questioning and open within a safe, containing environment.

A PERSONAL CASE EXAMPLE

The impact of being disbelieved must not be underplayed, nor can the communicative aspect of projective identification be undervalued. The following case example describes such a powerful personal experience that it is more accurately conveyed in the first person.

One of the women patients suddenly, and to my mind totally unexpectedly, called me a liar. At the time I was unable to identify why I was knocked out of kilter, but my reaction was that of a patient and not a professional nurse. My acting out took the form of virtually ignoring the patient until my thinking began to return. I felt very uncomfortable at the growing realization that we had swapped roles and it took some time to process what had happened. From this patient I felt some of the enormous pain and outrage that she had felt at being disbelieved as a child and gained some understanding of the extent of the pain experienced by the disbelieved child. In fact I very nearly retorted, when I was called a liar: 'It's not true, it's not fair, I didn't lie!'

PROJECTIVE IDENTIFICATION

My understanding of projection is that it is a form of communication, but it is also a technique of expelling unwanted parts of the self, in this case the patient, into the external object, in this case the nurse, primarily as a primitive defence mechanism; characteristics or desires that are unacceptable to a person's ego are externalized or projected onto someone else. Projective identification is a Kleinian concept (Hinshelwood 1989, 1994) which clarifies how the patient can push parts of their internal world, including anxieties and defences, into the recipient and this can become a method of controlling the object. The purpose of such an event can vary and, in addition to communication and control, can be a means of 'safeguarding the good self and/or good objects from the bad, getting rid of the bad internal objects, and empathy' (Solomon 1995, p.3). Projection is a deliberate action of which the projector is aware, whereby they imagine that specific impulses are located in an external object (Rycroft 1968), whilst both parties can be unaware of projective identification and the nurse can feel these emotions as their own and then unconsciously identify with the projected feelings. This state of mind is known as the counter-transference (Halton 1994) and the recipients of projective identification may often act out the counter-transference arising from the projected feeling. In projective identification the external object can become 'possessed by, controlled and identified with the projected parts' (Segal 1988, p.27). This is not to suggest that the object will now necessarily change, because the projection remains the phantasy of the patient, but nevertheless, it is of note that, for the patients we are thinking about, the appalling environment of their infancy and childhood has exacerbated and confirmed their sense that the external world is bad and emphasizes the omnipotence of their own malevolent phantasies. Consequently, the impact of projective identification on the organization as a whole, or on an individual within it, can be tremendous.

BEING UNBALANCED AND SUSPICIOUS OF SELF

The previous case example illustrated a moment when the communication of distress overwhelmed the nurse, but in an environment where active thinking is given a space the pain may be tolerated and processed and the patient provided with a place of containment wherein she can safely express herself. Within this safe, containing atmosphere communication has a place to develop. The development of psychodynamic practice within the team has allowed them to acknowledge inner disturbances resulting from the nature of their work. Without this acknowledgement and psychodynamic containment it is difficult to recognize the state of 'being unbalanced' and staff may then be unable to work through it and subsequently take refuge in fight or flight. Bion (1961) identifies these actions as being the only two techniques of self-preservation that an unthinking group seems to know. We do not work in isolation and, without psychodynamic thinking, may well become caught up in a group where the basic assumption is self-preservation of the group.

Menzies Lyth (1988) describes how confusion, both within the helping institutions and in society, as to what actually is the primary task of such organizations, leads to turmoil and anxiety. Bearing this in mind, it is not difficult to consider that such anxieties are exacerbated when the nurse is balancing the role of therapist and gaoler. Furthermore, society appears unsure of its feelings towards forensic mental health services and there is anecdotal indication that many people are more comfortable in a denial state of mind.

CONCLUSION: BENEVOLENT SUSPICION

It is hoped that this chapter has been able to illustrate the need for both suspicion and honesty, and the belief that this can be used to achieve safe empowerment for all. We need to value and support open and honest engagement in order to reduce the attack on care and to use this as a tool for empowering the patient to be successfully involved in planning their own care. Serious collusion occurs when neither nurse nor patient can integrate the needs of victim and perpetrator and this 'secret understanding' creates an obstruction that is left hanging in the therapeutic balance.

Maintaining benevolent and therapeutic suspicion is no easy task, especially within such toxic environments as illustrated earlier. However, clinical enquiry helps to validate such stressors. It is particularly important that we validate and share the difficulties in maintaining a balance and acknowledge that our own position shifts constantly. There are times when we are able to consciously observe unbalanced states of minds, but at others we are so caught up in the toxicity ourselves that we lose the capability of rational thought or indeed, on occasions, any thought and also the capacity to make sound judgements. Personal experience has suggested that it is useful, and rewarding, to practise to be constructively suspicious: that is, suspicious of both the feelings and actions of staff, including self, as well as our patients. It is arguably obvious that suspicion should not be malevolent or destructive, but should be undertaken with benevolent curiosity and a mindful wariness, in order to avoid suspicious stagnation and a consequential stalemate in therapeutic care. Finally, curiosity destroys repudiation and therefore curiosity may be suppressed as a defence. We have a need to develop the ability to tolerate not understanding and remain curious (and suspicious). But let us do this openly, *with* our patients, and empower a culture that can maintain a balance between care and custody, containment and control or even therapeutic engagement and liberal *laissez faire*.

REFERENCES

Aiyegbusi, A. (2001) 'Nursing Interventions and Future Directions with Women in Secure Services.' In Kettles, A., Woods, P. and Collins M. (eds) *Therapeutic Interventions for Forensic Mental Health Nurses*. London: Jessica Kingsley Publishers.

Aiyegbusi, A. (2004) 'Thinking under Fire: The Challenge for Forensic Mental Health Nurses Working with Women in Secure Care.' In Jeffcote, N. and Watson, T. (eds) *Working Therapeutically with Women in Secure Mental Health Settings*. London: Jessica Kingsley Publishers.

Bion, W.R. (1961) *Experiences in Groups*. London: Tavistock Publications Limited.

Department of Health (2002) *Women's Mental Health: Into the Mainstream. Strategic Development of Mental Health Care for Women*. London: HMSO.

Griffiths, P. and Leach, G. (1998) 'Psychosocial Nursing: A Model Learnt from Experience.' In Barnes, E., Griffiths, P., Ord, J. and Wells, D. (eds) *Face to Face with Distress: The Professional Use of Self in Psychosocial Care*. Oxford: Butterworth-Heinemann.

Halton, W. (1994) 'Some Unconscious Aspects of Organisational Life.' In Obholzer, A., and Roberts, V. (eds) *The Unconscious at Work: Individual and Organizational Stress in the Human Services* London: Routledge.

Hinshelwood, R.D. (1989) *A Dictionary of Kleinian Thought*. London: Free Association Books.

Hinshelwood, R.D. (1994) *Clinical Klein*. London: Free Association Books.

Hughes, L. and Pengelly, P. (1997) *Staff Supervision in a Turbulent Environment*. London: Jessica Kingsley Publishers.

Klein, M. (1959) 'Our Adult World and its Roots in our Infancy.' In *The Writings of Melanie Klein*. Vol.3. London: Hogarth Press and Institute of Psycho-Analysis, 1975.

Menzies Lyth, I. (1988) *Containing Anxiety in Institutions*. London: Free Association Books.

Roberts, V. (1994) 'The Organization at Work.' In Obholzer, A. and Roberts, V. (eds) *The Unconscious at Work*. London: Routledge.

Rycroft, C. (1968) *A Clinical Dictionary of Psychoanalysis*. 2nd edition. London: Penguin.

Segal, H. (1988) *Introduction to the Work of Melanie Klein*. London: Karnac Books.

Solomon, I. (1995) *A Primer of Kleinian Theory*. Northvale, NJ: Jason Aronson.

CHAPTER 14

A Secure Model of Nursing Care for Women

Jenifer Clarke-Moore and Miranda Barber

INTRODUCTION

This chapter will explore the challenges forensic nurses face when working with women in secure services and the need to develop an integrated model of nursing care based on the development of secure base behaviour.

The secure model of nursing care was developed as a result of confusion and sheer desperation in relation to attempts to work with a patient group that seemed largely unresponsive to the usual recognized approaches. The greatest challenge appeared to be an inability to provide compassionate, consistent care and instead becoming trapped in a culture of blame, splitting and scapegoating, with the patient being the most obvious scapegoat.

A research dissertation that explored nurses' experience of caring for women in a secure environment (Clarke 1999) concluded that the most fundamental problem confronting nurses was the lack of a coherent theoretical framework in relation to the complex interpersonal relationships that emerged when working with women in secure services. Whilst there were some similarities to the difficulties that were experienced when working with male patients, the levels of nurses' distress, frustration and despair when caring for women was considerably greater. It was also evident that the secure service we worked in appeared less successful with regard to care and treatment for women when compared to men, with more women being nursed on one-to-one observations for lengthy periods and a higher incidence of women being transferred to other secure services as placements broke down. The nurses also described feeling overwhelmed with having to continuously cope with high levels of 'acting-out' behaviour such as violence, self-harm and suicide attempts (Clarke 1999).

The conclusions of this research are in keeping with observations made within the National Women's Mental Health Strategy (Department of Health 2002), which highlighted the paucity of published research regarding models of care that specifically address women's needs. Women within secure services often experience extreme relationship difficulties which are often re-enacted, creating chaos in the system of care around them. This often results in women either being moved from one service to another or being detained for lengthy periods of time in services offering greater levels of physical security than are required.

As the title of this chapter suggests, 'A secure model of nursing care' is a nurse-led intervention; however, in order for it to be effective it requires a shared vision and understanding within the multidisciplinary approach.

THEORETICAL CONCEPT

Bowlby's theory of attachment considers an individual's significant relationships and their ongoing impact on the level of functioning. Bowlby proposes that if during childhood and adolescence the individual's primary care-givers are generally available, sensitive to their signals and consistently responsive, then that person develops confidence that supportive care is accessible (Bowlby 1969, 1973). These expectations are what is meant by a 'secure base' and allows both exploration of the environment and ease of soothing when distressed. In contrast, when care is unpredictable and highly conflictual, then an anxious attachment occurs. This can result in disruption to an individual's beliefs about themselves and others, leaving them vulnerable to expectations that others will not be able to successfully contain their emotional needs, and that they themselves are not worthy of care. Attachment theory also proposes that an individual will experience anxiety in response to the threat of, or actual separation from an attachment figure.

Examination of the background histories of many patients in secure services often brings to light instances in which the individual has experienced separation or threatened abandonment from significant others, for example threats of suicide by a parent. Not only do threats of abandonment create intense anxiety, but they also arouse anger, often of an intense degree. Those who are exposed to abuse or extreme forms of punishment are not only faced with threats to their attachment figure's availability, but must also manage a more profound dilemma when the attachment figure is also a source of danger.

ATTACHMENT STYLES

The clinical importance of the concept and theory of attachment is that once these principles are grasped there is less difficulty in understanding the complex interpersonal behaviours presented by women in secure care. Patients will react to carers based on their own attachment history. This is of particular importance for nurses who spend the longest periods of time with patients in secure settings and are most likely to be involved with the most intimate aspects of patients' care.

Those with a dismissing style may find it difficult to engage therapeutically, as they invest their energies in avoiding thinking about painful feelings. This is often interpreted by staff as failure to engage. It can also be demonstrated by excessive reliance on mind-altering substances such as illicit drugs or PRN (prescription required as needed) medication. In contrast, those with anxious ambivalent attachment styles tend to have an attachment system that is chronically hyper-activated. Attachment relationships to staff and other patients are often unstable, with rapid changes of mood and behaviour. Their frantic attempts to seek proximity and emotional fusion with carers can lead them being seen by clinical teams as demanding and emotionally draining. Individuals with this attachment style can also present with high levels of hostile, self-destructive and challenging behaviour, both as a way of engaging a care-giver interpersonally and to express anger and distress at perceived abandonment.

Once insecure attachment patterns are established, they are repeated, become more entrenched and more likely to operate outside conscious awareness. Patients will interact with others based on expectations and assumptions built from earlier relationships. Clinical staff need to identify and work constructively with these patterns. This is additionally complicated by the fact that staff do not come themselves as a 'blank slate' and will have their own attachment style. Adshead (2002) describes how staff teams frequently get caught up in the types of unhelpful attachment patterns described above and this often results in splits in staff teams.

Whilst this may lead to therapeutic despondency and pessimism, there is increasing evidence that dysfunctional attachment patterns can be altered through the experience of a psychodynamic understanding and emotional support. A containing consistent relationship will, over repeated interactions, challenge previous expectations and beliefs around disturbed attachment patterns. As women become more secure within the therapeutic milieu, they become more able to signal their needs clearly, and approach staff directly for help. They also begin to develop a secure sense of themselves as deserving of attention and support. The therapeutic relationship then allows a further purpose. The building of a secure base with the nursing team is a vital building block, allowing the person to engage in other therapeutic work with other disciplines (Barber *et al.* 2006).

PRACTICAL APPLICATION OF THE MODEL

Therapeutic communities have long used attachment theory as a model of care whilst working with people with personality disorders. However, despite there being a high incidence of women in secure services having either a primary or secondary diagnosis of personality disorder few services have attempted to integrate attachment theory within the therapeutic care package. A secure attachment model of nursing care for women can best be conceptualized in terms of the following stages:

Stage 1: Establishing a secure base

Whilst a whole systems approach is paramount the entire care package is dependent on whether or not the nursing team feels competent and confident in their ability to contain the patient safely. One of the difficulties previously experienced by ward-based nurses has been the failure of other disciplines to acknowledge the need to ensure that the nursing team feels adequately supported and confident to manage high-risk behaviours.

Case example

Ms C was transferred from an acute mental health unit to conditions of medium security having attempted to set fire to a litter bin. She had been in medium security for three months during which time there had been an increase in her self-harming behaviour and aggression to others. Ms C had a significant history of deprivation and trauma which included child sexual abuse and she described feeling increasingly distressed as a result of flashbacks of the abuse.

During these first three months Ms C had been allocated two primary nurses. The first had left shortly after Ms C's arrival and the second had been on long-term sick leave. Ms C had, however, engaged with a clinician who was working with her on her experiences of childhood sexual abuse. The clinical team became increasingly concerned as Ms C's self-harming behaviour was escalating and becoming life-threatening.

The nursing team was equally concerned and expressed anxieties about their ability to contain Ms C safely. They also reported an increase in high-risk behaviours following the sessions when Ms C had been making disclosure about the sexual abuse she experienced in childhood. The nursing team did not feel they had really got to know Ms C and her relationships with them had been generally superficial.

Ms C had difficulty articulating her feelings but was able to acknowledge that she felt lonely and believed this may have made the second of her primary nurses ill. She also disclosed that she was finding sessions looking at her child sexual abuse difficult but was reluctant to stop them as she desperately wanted the flashbacks to stop and she didn't want to upset her therapist.

Following a spate of physical assaults on nursing staff and further fire setting incidents it was agreed that Ms C could no longer be managed within the service and she was transferred to conditions of high security.

On reflection the impact of Ms C's early attachment relationships had not been clearly understood or taken into account which led to an inevitable re-enactment of her negative early life events. Ms C's mother had left the family home during Ms C's first few months of life and had not made any contact with the family since that time. Her father had remarried shortly afterwards; however, his new wife was diagnosed with cancer when Ms C was three years old. Ms C recalled her stepmother being extremely unwell for the following three years and she passed away when Ms C was six years old. She remembered being told to be 'good and not to cause her mother any worry'. Following the death of her stepmother Ms C was sent to stay with relatives during which time she was sexually abused by her older male cousins. Ms C tried to tell people what was happening to her which resulted in her being rejected by her relatives and eventually being placed in care when she was 12 years old. She had spent her entire adult life in various care settings, frequently being moved in response to difficulties containing her safely.

Ms C had no contact with her family despite many unsuccessful attempts on her part to do so. Her father was remarried, had a new family and did not want further contact with her. She had also tried unsuccessfully to contact her mother.

There were a number of issues that the team had failed to acknowledge:

- the impact of loss and abandonment of key figures involved in her care
- her fear of repercussions when disclosing her experiences of child sexual abuse
- her inability to cope with overwhelming emotions which were further triggered by the individual sessions to explore her experiences of child sexual abuse.

While Ms C had established a good relationship with the clinician who was doing the individual work with her, she described feeling she had nowhere to go after these sessions and was engulfed with intolerable emotions.

Implications for practice

If we consider Bowlby's (1969) perspective the building up of a more secure base will act as a building block, allowing patients to engage in multidisciplinary care and treatment programmes. On admission, patients are likely to be in crisis. Their mental state may be unstable and they will be dealing with transitional changes such as new relationships and alterations in environment, routines and expectations. At this point the primary focus of the clinical team is to stabilize the patient's mental state and establish a more secure relational base with the patient. The actual building of a secure base and awareness of the challenges to the patient's attachment expectations that this entails is the core intervention. The availability and responsiveness of clinical staff is also critical. However, it depends not only on the physical presence or absence of staff, but more importantly on the quality of the interactions. Staff have to be active in providing secure base support. In this process they need to be interested and open to detecting signals and recognizing distress, and be able to interpret correctly the need being communicated by the patient. In addition, staff need to be able to provide a timely, appropriate, cooperative response that supports and protects the well-being of the patient, within the boundaries of the therapeutic alliance.

Implementing a psychodynamic core team approach

Prior to admission, a fully comprehensive, multidisciplinary pre-admission assessment is completed. Potential disturbances in attachment status, such as previous splitting of clinical teams, can usually be anticipated via information gathered through clinical interview with the patient and existing carers, and through a review of available case notes.

Where there have been severely disrupted attachment patterns, a core nursing team is allocated to work alongside the primary nurse, to reduce the intensity of the transference and reduce the risk of damaging re-enactments. The core team has an in-depth knowledge of the patient, and works collaboratively to support each other in maintaining a consistent and empathic response, and in boundary maintenance. This is vital in assisting the nursing staff to tolerate the intensity of the patient's interpersonal dynamics.

A psychodynamic nursing core team is implemented for patients who experience significant relationship difficulties and have a history of problems receiving care within previous therapeutic relationships. While this could be argued as best practice for all patients there are significant resource implications and so patients' needs for core teams are prioritized.

As more members of the multiprofessional team become involved in the patient's care they are included within the core team. Reflective practice is mandatory for all core team members.

The value of core teams lies in:

- providing a coordinated, consistent approach to patients – aiding clearer communication, understanding and planning
- facilitating close multiprofessional working and early identification of problems
- having the potential to streamline clinical team meetings, such as CPAs (Care Programme Approach), by selecting information that needs to be discussed. Detailed exploration of the patient's internal world and team dynamics are explored in more depth in core team meetings
- ensuring care plans are multiprofessionally developed, refined and evaluated

- providing a framework and secure base for all team members that protect clinicians from working in isolation and experiencing burnout
- reducing the risk of clinicians becoming drawn into re-enactments of prior negative experiences and relationships with care-givers.

Stage 2: Maintaining a secure base and supporting recovery

Commitment to attending group reflective practice, by both qualified and unqualified staff, is imperative to the implementation of this model. These sessions allow a thinking space to focus on understanding the patient's internal world, and understanding how past traumas can be re-enacted. This understanding helps to counter malignant alienation, which can result in the clinical team becoming disjointed in their thinking around a patient's care, and deeply divided in their responses between displays of hostility and empathy. The process of reflection assists with effective risk assessment and management, and helps the team to work proactively, rather than purely reactively.

Stage 3: Maintenance of a secure base through discharge and follow-up

The need to maintain relational security to manage risk becomes particularly apparent at the stage of discharge and after-care. As the secure base becomes more internalized within the patient, she becomes empowered to function more independently, and her self-esteem and confidence increase. This may be complicated by any fluctuations in the patient's mental health and emotional well-being, which may lead to an underestimation of the level of emotional support required to sustain progress.

The capacity of women in secure services to manage issues related to their risk is dependent on a variety of factors. However, it is feasible to assume that the level of disruption within the attachment system may have important predictive powers with regard to risk of relapse and recidivism. Those with more disrupted and incoherent attachment patterns may be at particular risk of reverting back to previous, more maladaptive attachment strategies at times of transition, when they experience actual or threatened separations from significant care-givers. For these patients successful ongoing management of their pathway out of secure care may be more significantly related to the level of relational security provided by a placement and care team than the level of procedural security around them.

CONCLUSION

The behaviours of women in secure services are frequently described as chaotic and 'non-understandable'. Attachment theory underpins the development of a practical model of nursing care, which addresses the diverse presentations and psychopathologies demonstrated by these women. The theoretical framework assists in the understanding of the relevance of early, disrupted attachments, which are subsequently re-enacted, and informs the development of clinical interventions which are meaningful both to the individual women and the clinical team working with them.

REFERENCES

Adshead, G. (2002) 'Three degrees of security: Attachment and forensic institutions.' *Criminal Behaviour and Mental Health 12*, 2, 31–45.

Barber, M., Short, J., Clarke-Moore, J., Lougher, M., Huckle, P. and Amos, T. (2006) 'A secure attachment model of care: Meeting the needs of women with mental health problems and antisocial behaviour.' *Criminal Behaviour and Mental Health* 16, 3–10.

Bowlby, J. (1969) *Attachment and Loss Volume 1: Attachment.* London: Penguin Books.

Bowlby, J. (1973) *Attachment and Loss Volume 2: Separation: Anxiety and Anger.* London: Penguin Books.

Clarke, J. (1999) 'Nurses' experience of working with women in a mixed sex secure service.' Unpublished MSc thesis, Middlesex University/Tavistock Clinic.

Department of Health (2002) *Women's Mental Health Strategy: Into the Mainstream. Strategic Department of Mental Health Care for Women.* London: Department of Health.

CHAPTER 15

Working with One Another: Service User/Professional

Joanne Roberts and Jenifer Clarke-Moore

INTRODUCTION

As health care professionals we spend much of our time (with the best of intentions) planning, implementing and evaluating care. While we try to involve patients as much as possible in this process we rarely have the opportunity to later reflect with our patients their experience of the care they have received and our experience of caring for them. We have as much to learn from one another as we do from our standard ways of learning.

We have been in the privileged position of having worked together for over 15 years and have since attempted to share and reflect on our experiences. This chapter will tell our story as we experienced it so we fully accept that others may have different views and perceptions.

JO

I was a student nurse just starting the second year of my training. It had been a difficult journey to get to this point having experienced a lot of trauma and disruption in my early life, spending periods in care and missing a lot of schooling. I'd had to work hard to be accepted for nurse training.

At the age of 19 I would describe myself as 'full of life' and a 'bit of a party animal'. Things started to go wrong when I was on holiday with a group of other student nurses in Magaluf and one night in an intoxicated state I was apparently 'ballet dancing' on the balcony when I fell off and knocked myself out for a couple of seconds. I still don't know if this had anything to do with what happened next but everything seemed to go wrong from that point.

About two weeks after returning from the holiday I started to feel 'strange', sort of paranoid, and that developed into derogatory voices which I didn't feel able to tell anyone about and couldn't make sense of myself. I started drinking heavily to stop the voices and consumed up to a bottle of vodka a day just to be able to sleep. I impulsively took an overdose, because I wanted 'everything to go away'. Everything becomes a bit blurred at this point but I ended up in the accident and emergency department of my local hospital. I remember waking up to find nurses and doctors at the bottom of the bed and thought they were laughing and talking about me. I still have no recollection of what happened next but was told that I had seriously assaulted a nurse and had made threats to kill. I still don't really know about the details of this assault and think that maybe there is a part of me that would rather not know. If someone had told me that I'd put a bomb under parliament at that time I wouldn't be able to deny it; I had no idea what was going on.

Attempts were made to find me a hospital bed but there was nothing available at that time so I was remanded to prison. After a few weeks I was sent to an independent secure service and was placed on a teenage behavioural unit, where it seemed to me that everyone was running riot. I remember there being a point system, which I never really understood. I kept losing points and couldn't understand why. I didn't see my family for a year and telephone contact was limited because of the point system. On a positive note the day was very structured which meant the time went quickly and there were things to do. In a matter of months my life had been transformed from having responsibility, power and choice to being totally controlled by others. I was still experiencing confusing thoughts and beliefs and found it impossible to make sense of what was going on around me.

I was eventually assessed and accepted by a new medium secure service, which was in my home town. I recall being the first patient to be admitted which meant that I got an incredible amount of attention from staff, which was very different to where I had come from. In fact many of the nursing staff seeming more like friends to me. The surroundings were also totally different, more luxurious, but maybe the greatest difference was that there was no structure to the day. This meant I spent most of my time sitting around chatting to staff.

JEN

This brings us to the point when I met Jo. I was a newly appointed charge nurse for the intensive care unit. Jo was the first patient I was introduced to and I immediately sensed some unease within myself which I initially put this down to first-day nerves. I tried to apply what I thought were my reasonably effective communication skills to strike up some conversation which appeared to really irritate Jo: so much in fact that she began to pace back and forth. I was advised to go in the ward office and stay there. My recollection of that meeting was of feeling as though my heart was thumping in my throat, being totally inadequate, de-skilled and wondering what on earth I'd done coming to the job. On reflection I had been ambushed by a powerful projective identification in that Jo's persecutory ideations had reverberated with my own sense of vulnerability. Without a theoretical framework to make sense of what was happening I felt completely out of my depth. I sensed the institutional pressure to be a 'good nurse' in the eyes of others, a sort of 'ideal mother' rather than a 'good enough nurse'. I felt I had failed miserably. With hindsight, I see that what was happening is well explained by Tom Main (1989) in his paper entitled 'The ailment', with the 'in-group' and the 'out group'. On the ward, those nurses who could work with Jo were seen to be more experienced and knowledgeable. Those whom Jo seemed to dislike were seen as unable to work with her and therefore less able as nurses.

The following day I found myself moved to another ward which actually reinforced my fears and feelings of inadequacy. On reflection I took Jo's rejection quite personally and was relieved not to have to go back. What I hadn't been prepared for was that I was going to experience a similar response during my initial attempts to interact with other patients and I would say more specifically it was extremely difficult to strike up a rapport with the women patients. Again this was very different to my experiences of working as a nurse in acute mental health settings. While I was aware of the dilemma faced by forensic nurses in attempting to be nurturing as well as being in a position of control I was at this point totally unaware of how people carry with them their own internal institutions, families and patterns of behaviour which they project onto others (Killian and Clark 1996).

I have since discussed my experience of our first meeting with Jo who had no recollection of it but she does remember feeling scared when new people came onto the ward.

JO

I remember this being a difficult time when it never seemed clear what I was expected to do and that the goal posts seemed to change all the time. For example, if I self-harmed, sometimes I would find my ground leave stopped and other times staff would take me out on leave. I had no idea what was going on and how decisions were being made; it seemed to depend more on who was in charge rather than what I did. Some events really impacted on me, like having my primary nurse changed suddenly and not being told the reason for this. I was convinced that I must have done something wrong. Another incident that sticks in my mind was when I had to see a psychotherapist for an assessment. I found the assessment extremely intrusive and the psychotherapist even got important facts wrong which made me really cross. I remember feeling so angry that I smashed up the entire contents of the kitchen. While I was clearly unwell for much of this time there were incidents that enraged me that were not linked to illness but more to do with being treated with a total lack of respect. There seemed to be all sorts of attempts at new therapies such as psychodrama which actually left me feeling more traumatized. One minute I'd be socializing with staff and the next I'd be having some kind of therapy which I didn't understand. My self-harming was also confusing. Sometimes I would cut myself just to reassure myself that I wasn't an alien but sometimes I did it to get attention and sometimes I'd just had enough and wanted it all to end. This was really difficult to describe to anyone.

I felt as if everything was spiralling out of control and was put on more and more medication. Then there would be days and weeks of special observations and long periods in restraint. My recollection of this is still one of fear and horror and I remember feeling not only that my mind was out of control but that suddenly I had no control over my body. Some time later I was told that I was going to be put on a behaviour programme. This was probably the most punishing and painful experience of all. It was as if everyone thought I was doing things to get at them. Suddenly everyone was treating me differently. Nurses I thought I got on well with suddenly stopped talking to me. It felt like I had to do something wrong to get attention. Again my thoughts were getting more confused and fuzzy. I then seriously assaulted a member of staff whom I'd previously had a good relationship with. Again I have no recollection of this other than that I thought I was going to be forcibly medicated. Following this incident, I was transferred to a high security psychiatric hospital and I remember being absolutely petrified.

There was little to no furniture on the high security psychiatric ward. I was nursed on a ward for patients with personality disorder. I saw patients cutting one another and I was afraid to go to the toilets in case I found someone hanging, which was a usual occurrence. I was glad to be locked in my room at night just to know I was safe. I believe the positive side of being there was the people believing and understanding that I had little control over my thoughts and subsequent actions at that time. The clinical team decided to put me on Clozaril which I believe changed my life. I also developed a good therapeutic relationship with my male primary nurse who had a belief in me. I was also having regular contact with my home team from the medium secure unit. I thought I was going to be forgotten but they constantly reassured me that this was a short-term placement. Without that sense of hope I'm not sure I would have survived.

JEN

The decision to send any patient to a high security psychiatric hospital is frequently fraught with difficulties and differences of opinions. On reflection, we were a new enthusiastic medium secure service and there was an eagerness to try new therapies and approaches to care, but this was coupled with inexperienced staff and the absence of a coherent theoretical framework to guide us with regard to the complexity of Jo's needs. Some senior clinical staff had received training in forensic psychotherapy but generally there was a lack of understanding about the complexities that can emerge within the therapeutic relationship, for example, suddenly changing the primary nurse without considering Jo's attachment history and relationship needs. Also, there was no recognition of the need to take account of the risks of becoming embroiled in re-enactments of her negative early life experiences.

Whilst I had little input with Jo's care until this point I had started to develop an interest into why women appeared to do less well within medium security when compared with their male counterparts and I started to follow up those women who had been transferred to high security psychiatric hospitals. I wanted to try to understand how they had experienced their care with us and what we needed to do differently to ensure that we did not repeat any anti-therapeutic patterns when they returned to us. In clinical interviews with these women, common themes emerged which included not feeling safe, feeling confused about their relationships with staff, and having to engage in therapies they did not feel they could cope with or understand. This again seemed to replicate many of their early life experiences particularly for those patients who had experienced previous abuse and trauma.

I remember meeting what felt to be a very different Jo when I visited her in the high security psychiatric hospital. She appeared incredibly fragile, almost like an abandoned child. She was desperate to return to our service but wanted things to be different. There were very mixed feelings about Jo returning to our service. Members of the team who had kept in contact with Jo in the high security psychiatric hospital were convinced of the progress she had made and felt she was ready to move back. Those who worked closely with Jo previously and had become traumatized by the whole experience were understandably anxious about her impending return. As a team though, we knew we had to have a different approach to her care and treatment from the one we had in place prior to her transfer to the high security psychiatric hospital. We decided to implement what later became recognized as a core team nursing approach. The core team was identified prior to Jo's return and a number of preparatory meetings were held where issues of perceived difficulty were explored and discussed. While the core team was still led by a primary nurse who coordinated the care, the other members were just as involved in Jo's day-to-day care. This approach aimed to ensure consistency and to protect nurses from burnout by diluting the intensity of the transference. As a result of this approach, relationships felt less intense and more contained. The rationale behind this was that if you have a contained staff group, there is a greater chance of offering the patient containment and safety.

There had been a tendency within mental health generally to try to work on the causative factors of the disturbance rather than focusing on developing healthier functioning. For example, if a patient had a history of sexual abuse it was often the primary focus of the therapeutic intervention. There is sufficient evidence to suggest that this is not always in the best interest of the patient, particularly if they do not have the emotional resources to cope with the emotional distress that such sensitive work can provoke in them. Linehan's (1993) dialectical behaviour therapy model is an example of an intervention where the trauma isn't actively worked on until the high risk behaviours can be safely managed.

The core team was initially made up of a small group of experienced nursing staff and other disciplines who were involved in Jo's day-to-day care. Initially the core team received weekly psychodynamic reflective practice where Jo's internal world and the staff group's emotional responses were explored and thought about. So whilst we didn't apply a psychodynamic model in our direct clinical work with Jo, our increased understanding of her internal world and the emotional impact on staff enabled us to work in a more thoughtful, proactive manner. The treatment approach became more 'goal focused' rather than reactive and we all felt we were heading in the same direction. Importantly, by applying thought in this way, we were able to avoid becoming drawn into the sort of anti-therapeutic acting out that was evident in Jo's first admission to our service.

JO

My experiences on returning to the clinic were very different from my first admission. An important difference was that this time I knew what the goals of my care were. It was not all plain sailing though. After I had developed a positive relationship with my primary nurse she left, but this time it was talked about, explored and prepared for. I didn't think it had such a huge impact on my care for two reasons: I was more in control of my thoughts as a result of appropriate medication and I had already developed good relationships with other members of the core team. I must add at this point, that throughout all of this time the one constant was my RMO (responsible medical officer) who I felt always treated me as an equal, with respect and compassion and even during my most difficult times always seemed to have a belief in me. I continued to experience some break-through symptoms of my illness but now found that staff responded in a caring manner rather than constantly challenging and questioning me as to whether I was 'really' feeling paranoid and scared, and accepting what I told them.

I found moving into the community a challenging experience and found myself at loggerheads with the team for a while. The team was keen that I should live somewhere where there would be some level of care but I'd had enough of living with other people and wanted the chance to live in my own flat.

JEN

I can remember feeling a bit unnerved by the suggestion that Jo wanted to live independently and wasn't at all convinced that she had the skills to do so. I also knew Jo well enough by this point to know that unless she was signed up to any care plan it wasn't going to happen. We were fortunate to have a good team and we set about making the plan work. I'm convinced that this would never have become a reality if we hadn't been able to work together. Jo was followed up in the community by our forensic team for approximately two years and then her care was handed over to the local community mental health team. This followed a period of 12 months joint working between both the forensic and local community mental health teams. Jo and I did not have any contact for approximately four years after she had been transferred to the care of the local community mental health team. She continued to make progress in the community and I moved to pastures new.

I was extremely fortunate to have the opportunity to be involved in developing a new secure service for women in the independent sector. I guess this is one of the main highlights of my career, where working with a dynamic team with a supportive management structure made me feel that anything was possible. When it came to thinking about advocacy we agreed that if possible it should be someone who had actually experienced care in a secure service previously. There were a few of us in the service who had cared for Jo previously and felt she would be very effective in the role of advocate for other women receiving secure care. We gave careful thought to how this would be managed before we approached Jo to see if she was interested. It was vital that we could adapt our previous relationships and work with Jo as a colleague rather than a patient. This meant moving from a paternalist role to one of real equality. As much as we say we see our patients as equals and as individuals, we can sometimes become so hung up on maintaining the boundaries that the relationship is unable to move on and mature. I believe Jo and I were able to develop our relationship which evolved so that we were able to work together in partnership.

JO

I felt that being offered the advocacy job was a bigger achievement than being accepted for my nurse training. I felt like I was being given a second chance. I have been working as an advocate for approximately seven years and I believe my experiences as a service user have enabled me to offer hope to those I work with.

My final message for this chapter is that as long as hope is kept alive and someone believes in you then you can succeed regardless of anything else.

CONCLUSION

Jo found herself in a secure physical environment that isolated and to an extent alienated her from society. Her mental state exacerbated this sense of isolation. Being the first patient on the medium secure unit, Jo had few if any peers and her only human contact to a large extent were nurses, those 'paid to be friends'. Decisions about where she lived and what human interaction she had and with whom were out of her control.

The nature of nursing, the nurses' ongoing contact with the patient, the style of intervention and need to care can arouse intense counter-transference feelings. Of the multiprofessional clinical team, nurses are usually the ones who are required to force patients to take medication against their will, engage in special observations and on occasions use restraint. Taking this into account it is no wonder that nurses are perceived by the patient as being either 'good carers' or 'bad carers'. Additionally there is a professional expectation that nurses will engage with their patients, gaining their confidence and developing relationships that facilitate disclosure by the patient of their private lives. In doing so, nurses run the risk of projecting unwanted aspects of themselves into the patient and patient group. It is therefore a significant challenge to nursing to find ways that can prevent the development of unhealthy symbiotic relationships. This challenge can best be met by having a coherent theoretical framework and a comprehensive clinical supervision structure which was applied in this example by using psychodynamic reflective practice.

People we work with are human beings with the same frailties, misunderstandings, misinterpretations, misrepresentations and fears that we all have, except that theirs may be more intense and disabling. Regardless of how well meaning the staff around them might be there are real possibilities that patients are further traumatized and distressed by organizational behaviour and limitations. The technology that we practise with does not involve machines or equipment that goes bleep; we work with human technology in the form of our selves. It is our responsibility to learn, rehearse and reflect on how we work with both the individual patient and the organization that we are part of.

REFERENCES

Killian, M. and Clark, N. (1996) 'The Nurse.' In Cordess, C. and Cox, M. (eds) *Forensic Psychotherapy: Crime Psychodynamics and the Offender Patient.* 2 vols. London: Jessica Kingsley Publishers.

Linehan, M. (1993) *Cognitive Behavioural Treatment of Borderline Personality Disorder.* New York: The Guilford Press.

Main, T. (1989) 'The Ailment.' In *The Ailment and Other Psychoanalytic Essays.* London: Free Association Books.

CHAPTER 16

Loss and the Adolescent Offender

Maria McMillan

INTRODUCTION

The following chapter relates to some aspects of working as a forensic community mental health nurse (FCMHN) within a Youth Offending Team (YOT). This nursing post is a secondment from the Child and Adolescent Mental Health Services (CAMHS). The YOT provides a statutory service to children and adolescents aged between ten years and 18 years who have come into contact with the criminal justice system.

THE SETTING

The YOT comprises of workers from a variety of agencies and disciplines. Social workers and probation officers hold casework responsibility and work alongside police officers, teachers, youth workers, drugs workers and mental health workers in an effort to identify and address the practical and developmental needs of the young person or adolescent. The aim is to use the initial assessment of need and risk as a basis for formulating a plan which will support the adolescent to avoid further offending behaviour. The adolescent often presents with a complex and distressing history of having been failed by a series of environments: the primary carer, the family, the school and the community. The stories which unfold as the adolescent participates in the assessments can be painful and difficult to hear. Consequently, the caseworkers are constantly faced with the dilemma of having to attend to the welfare of the adolescent whilst also addressing their offending behaviour and ensuring punishment is administered.

Following on from the initial assessment and depending on outcomes, the caseworker can refer to colleagues in the team for specialist assessments of specific concerns such as substance misuse, dyslexia, emotional and mental health problems. There are three criteria for a referral to the mental health nurse. These are a history of self-harming behaviours, subjective or objective signs of psychiatric disturbance, or previous contact with mental health services. The criteria for referral are discerned through the use of standard questions set by the Youth Justice Board (the YOT's governing body), and are included in the initial generic assessment. However, referrals to the mental health nurse can also be motivated by the unbearable anxieties provoked in the caseworker through their contact with adolescents who present with difficulties ranging from withdrawn states to actively aggressive and dangerous behaviours. This is evidenced in the number of times 'bereavement issues' or 'anger management difficulties' are cited as the reasons for referral. Consequently, in receiving a referral the nurse becomes involved in a hidden task which is to emotionally contain the worker whilst considering the emotional and mental health needs of the young client.

Before thinking about the emotional demands of the nursing role I would like to add a comment about the parallel between the setting of the YOT and the hospital ward as observed by Menzies Lyth (1959). Before the adolescent is seen by the mental health nurse the caseworker has had to complete several forms, enter data into the computer system and measure the severity of particular problems in the process of ensuring most areas of the adolescent's life are considered. This enables the task of thinking about the complexity and discomfort of the adolescent's situation to be broken down into smaller, more manageable doses. As Menzies Lyth explains, this ensures the worker is prevented from 'coming effectively into contact with the totality of any one patient...and offers some protection from the anxiety this arouses' (p.51). So, at the point of referral the nurse potentially represents a container for all the 'messy' emotional aspects of the adolescent's world which impede the progress of the caseworker's duties. An awareness of this dynamic is crucial so that the nurse can recognize these projections as stemming from the referrer's anxiety and so avoid becoming identified with the unbearable aspects of the adolescent.

THE ADOLESCENT PROCESS

In an emotionally contained environment, anxiety could be viewed as a valid and necessary reaction to the adolescent offender. Winnicott (1964) considers the troubling and disturbing behaviours of delinquents as an attempt by the adolescent to mobilize action in the adult world by generating anxiety. By re-framing the adolescent's antisocial behaviour anybody who works therapeutically with them is enabled to see themselves as a hopeful, positive participant in the adolescent's life, especially as the case-worker, identified with authority, is imbued with parental associations. The relevance to this setting is that the adolescent offender's unconscious wish for such a figure is complicated by their developmental need to separate from their parents and they are inevitably parents with whom the adolescent has a very chaotic and damaged attachment to. Anna Freud (1967) describes the confusion of ambivalent feelings towards the parents at this stage of growing up:

> It is normal for an adolescent to behave...in an inconsistent manner; to love his parents and hate them; to revolt against them and to be dependent on them; to be deeply ashamed to acknowledge his mother before others and, unexpectedly, to desire heart-to-heart talks with her. (p.275)

Adolescents who are busy with the age-appropriate task of questioning their parents' authority also have to relinquish their world-view which held them together during latency. The loss of certainty about their parents and about themselves in relation to their parents, stirs up anxieties during the period of adolescence. Freud (1926) made the link between loss and anxiety when he described how the loss of the object causes an accumulation of unsatisfied needs, desires and wishes. These frustrations provoke a sense of helplessness which requires defending against in order for the adolescent to survive psychically. In the case of the adolescent offender, the defence often adopted against the anxiety of feeling helpless is to project the feeling onto a 'victim' in the context of a violent act.

Often, the response from society via the criminal justice system comes in the form of a good enough YOT intervention. When the court sentences the adolescent to a community penalty they will be seen weekly by a case-worker and be expected to fulfil a number of requirements such as reparation, all of which can be perceived as a form of benign attention, despite also being a punishment. For severely deprived or traumatized adolescents, this form of attention can have a paradoxical effect. The risk is that appointments to see the caseworker become a re-enactment of an earlier abusive relationship with an adult. The interviews with drugs workers or mental health workers are perceived as a form of humiliation and hence to be avoided. Whatever is offered is rejected as it is a concrete reminder of earlier losses and deprivations. Such adolescents are problematic and thwart the numerous tasks the caseworker is expected to fulfil. Consequently the caseworker's defences against anxiety are breached and they are exposed to painful feelings and projections of helplessness which emanate from the adolescent.

The paucity of opportunity to consider the emotional impact of youth justice work often leads to the need for this aspect of the work to be displaced onto the nurse. Freidman and Laufer (1997) describe the process which occurs in work with disturbed adolescents: 'our anxiety to do something about a crisis...may in fact be due to being made to feel by the adolescent that his tension is unbearable, and not because there is any action that we can usefully undertake'. It is important for the nurse to be conscious of this process and to respect how such tensions confound casework culture. By holding this in mind the nurse begins to contribute towards a containing environment.

CASE STUDY 1

The following study describes the effect on a traumatized boy of receiving a community order programme following his first offence. The impact on the nurse of the ensuing dynamics between colleagues will be explored.

Shaun was a 16-year-old boy who had narrowly avoided a custodial sentence. A psychiatric court report had recommended contact with CAMHS as a condition of Shaun's community order. He had a history of serious self-harming ideas and acts which were connected to the death of his mother some years earlier. He had a family who could not attend to his needs as they themselves had been traumatized by his mother's death and consequently overlooked Shaun's gradual withdrawal from them, his school and friends over two years. Shaun's offence was armed robbery during which he had held a knife to his victim's throat. Shaun was very quickly startled by the victim's retaliation and aborted his attempt at robbery. When the police arrived at the scene they found Shaun in a regressed state, sobbing and trembling.

In the course of my work with Shaun, I had noticed a huge disparity between his verbal precocity and the feelings he induced in me which suggested he was very dependent on our contact. He would arrive early for our appointments and, despite initial protests that he did not need to see me, Shaun had difficulty leaving the sessions and always left me with feelings of profound hopelessness and the anxiety that he might resume his self-harming behaviours. This anxiety was partly orchestrated by Shaun and I came to understand it as a re-enactment of the sadistic qualities which had briefly but powerfully emerged in the offence.

Shaun's caseworker Helen had a different emotional experience of him and was frequently exasperated by him. He failed to cooperate with the several plans she had put in place for him. In her irritation with Shaun, Helen often challenged my intervention, as though questioning why I was not making him 'better' and more motivated. There was a split between us which Shaun effectively promoted. I was being idealized by him as the one who would listen and respond sensitively, while Helen was seen as the bully who was trying to organize his life. She was trying in earnest to make sure Shaun was reintegrated into some form of structure and gainful activity. Helen finally learned from Shaun that he enjoyed music. After much effort and initiative Helen managed to gain access to funding from a local youth project in order to buy Shaun a guitar. They had discussed it and he promised he would join a music class once he had the guitar.

When Helen triumphantly presented the guitar to Shaun he refused to take it. He claimed there were faults with it and objected to the model, the size and the tone. This was too much for Helen to bear and she threatened to breach his community order and return him to court. According to the expectations of his community order, Shaun had failed to comply. My task as his nurse was to think of Shaun's refusal to cooperate as a communication. Helen and I were being drawn into acting out the roles of significant people in Shaun's mind which was evidently profoundly split. This was projected into the workers and it deepened the split between Helen's role and my own. I experienced her attempts to engage Shaun as intrusive and insensitive, while she perceived my involvement with him as 'precious' and indulgent.

When I saw Shaun a few days later, he described feeling physically unable to take the guitar from Helen. I could sense the abhorrence in him as he said, 'Does she think I'm a charity case?' The guitar and Helen's efforts to make things better for him had been an embarrassing and painful reminder of how he had had to look after himself for so long. He could not tolerate the exposure of being seen as lacking something. This undermined the huge effort he had made in denying the loss of his mother and the inability of his family to consider his needs.

After expressing his indignation Shaun's affect changed and he put a poignant question to me: 'If I did take the guitar, what will I have to do to repay her?' In this comment Shaun was transformed from an outraged, obstinate youth to a frightened boy who had had no experience of being given something unconditionally. I felt moved by this honest expression of fear and suddenly gained insight into the extent of his early deprivation. I was also concerned how I might communicate my hypothesis about Shaun's earlier behaviour to Helen.

In considering my role in relation to this case and in trying to function effectively as a container, I needed to consider what I represented to both Shaun and Helen. Helen works in a system which does not provide space for thought. Her need for cooperation from Shaun was fuelled by her own unconscious motives, as is the case for all of us who work in the 'caring professions'. As with nurses on hospital wards, job satisfaction comes in the guise of seeing a client 'get better'. The adolescent who offends and 'refuses' to improve his behaviour causes frustration and anxiety which is then defended against. In this case the defence was a denial of the reality of Shaun's severely damaged sense of himself. The defence also manifested as a manic need to do something which would make him change. Although my sessions with Shaun initially served the purpose of containing the despair he presented with, paradoxically I became something to be envied. Helen imagined the contact I had with Shaun to be more rewarding than the contact she had with Shaun. To some extent this was based on a reality, as I was being supported through clinical supervision and was, in turn, being emotionally contained. The situation left me with the polarized experience of having to hold the anxiety of Shaun's potential risk to himself and to others, alongside the omnipotent feeling that I was something to be envied in the team.

Helen and I finally found a way of talking about how Shaun was affecting us. After all, Shaun's idealization of me left me vulnerable to being denigrated by him at some stage in the future. The improved communication between us made Shaun's attempts to split us more manageable. In turn, this gave him the experience of being thought about both as a deeply hurt boy and as a young adult who could perpetrate acts of violence.

I hope that the experience of having his emotional world acknowledged, but then not having the splits within it projected back to him, gave Shaun the beginnings of a more integrated sense of himself.

CASE STUDY 2

The next example is one in which the adolescent's experience of loss at an early age contributed to a very different use of the forensic mental health nurse's role.

Shah was 15 years old when he was convicted of robbery for which he received a custodial sentence. The victim of Shah's offence was a lone young woman. Immediately prior to his release from custody, Shah made a serious attempt to kill himself. The institution he was placed in did not have mental health services on site. His caseworker in the YOT requested that I visit him. We agreed that he required assessment for treatment in the community as part of his licence. When I arrived at the prison for our first meeting I was greeted by a probation officer who said that Shah was refusing to see me. I was concerned that he might have been too depressed to leave his cell. However, I was informed that my appointment clashed with Shah's scheduled session at the gym, which he was not prepared to miss. This communication from Shah set the tone for my subsequent contact with him. I felt ridiculous having travelled so far to see him only to be snubbed. I was also puzzled by the fact that staff had conceded to him, despite the very alarming behaviour which had triggered the referral to me. I decided it had been important for him to know that someone continued to think about the despair he had experienced some days before.

Once in the community and on licence, Shah and I managed to engage in regular contact. As a result, I began to understand his behaviour during my initial attempt to meet with him in custody. Born in Pakistan, he had been separated from his mother when aged five years. He remembered in vivid detail the scene of their separation. His father had brought him to this country as he thought Shah would have a better education which would bring with it better life chances. Shah had not seen his mother since that time and his father died soon after their arrival to this country. The pathos of his story and the trauma of Shah's history was moving, but I still held in mind the feeling he had provoked in me at the first visit when I felt annoyed at his refusal to see me; one of humiliation.

Shah would often say to me, 'I'm not being funny Miss, but all you do is sit there'. This comment resonated with the image I had of his mother who had allowed her son to be taken away and had proven ineffectual in preventing an unbearable event from happening. I also wondered whether this was his way of telling me he felt listened to but was unable to be explicit as that would imply his need and desire to feel listened to.

Shah's complaints about seeing me were freely expressed to my colleague John, Shah's caseworker. John would regularly mention to me that Shah was objecting to our appointments. I felt as if I was being mildly ridiculed by John and it occurred to me how Shah was managing the conflict of needing to talk but then feeling shame about revealing his vulnerability. Despite the apparent denigration of my work with Shah, John regularly reinforced to him the importance of continuing to see me. Perhaps this was an unconscious attempt on John's part to protect his capacity to continue with his duties.

Gradually, through our discussions John and I managed to reach an agreement that my sessions with Shah should continue. Consequently, Shah had the experience of John as validating his need to express painful feelings to me. We hoped that the validation may have brought about a less denigrating and aggressive attitude towards vulnerable women and towards aspects of himself of which he felt deeply ashamed. My role as nurse had been to experience the humiliating feelings in order to consider and understand them. Bearing such feelings was painful, but working with Shah felt important as he showed an eagerness to communicate.

In our last session, Shah spoke of his improved sense of self-control and his more satisfying relationships with peers at college. He said, 'It's amazing what talking can do!'

CONCLUSION

In the adolescent with a good enough early childhood the grieving for lost stability and routine which featured in latency can provoke a temporary disturbance. The residual memory of something safe and good gives hope and acts as a protective factor when the development of a sexual body and internal conflicts bring with them intense new feelings and a sense of loss (Horne 2000). In the cases I have described above, the boys had experienced accumulative, traumatic losses in early childhood. For such adolescents the 'normal' disturbance of adolescence can feel catastrophic. There is very little to fall back on emotionally, so the sense of falling apart is evacuated into someone else as an attempt to regain a sense of self. The adolescent offender may learn this as a device for alleviating emotional pain and so begin to depend on it habitually as a persistent offender. By coming to the attention of the YOT the adolescent offender unconsciously accesses the practical and emotional resources which evaded them previously and which could become a protective factor against continued offending. Whether the adolescent can then use the resources offered depends on the sensitivity and understanding with which they are delivered.

For the forensic nurse working in a community setting which is multi-agency, such as a YOT, their role involves considering emotional containment on several levels; not just in the work with the adolescent but also in the contact with colleagues in the team, and with external agencies. The forensic nurse's ultimate aim is that the adolescent's painful reality should not be avoided or denied, but be felt, tolerated and then, I hope, understood.

REFERENCES

Freidman, M.H. and Laufer, M.E. (1997) 'Problems in Working with Adolescents.' In Laufer, M.E. (ed.) *Adolescent Breakdown and Beyond.* London: Karnac.

Freud, S. (1926) *Inhibitions, Symptoms and Anxiety.* Standard Edition, Vol. 20. London: Hogarth.

Freud, A. (1967) 'Adolescence.' *The Psychoanalytic Study of the Child 13*, 255–78.

Horne, A. (2000) 'Normal Emotional Development.' In Lanyado, M. and Horne, A. (eds) *The Handbook of Child and Adolescent Psychotherapy.* London: Routledge.

Menzies Lyth, I. (1959) 'The Functioning of Social Systems as a Defence against Anxiety.' In Menzies Lyth, I. *Containing Anxiety in Institutions: Selected Essays*, Vol. 1. London: Free Association Books.

Winnicott, D.W. (1964) *The Child, the Family and the Outside World.* London: Penguin.

List of Contributors

John Adlam is Principal Adult Psychotherapist at Henderson Hospital Services and Group Psychotherapist at the St George's Eating Disorders Service at Springfield Hospital. He is also honorary lecturer in Forensic Psychotherapy, St George's University of London and is currently Vice President of the International Association for Forensic Psychotherapy.

Gwen Adshead is a forensic psychiatrist and forensic psychotherapist. For the past ten years she has been Consultant Forensic Psychotherapist in Broadmoor Hospital. She is a group analyst and also has an interest in attachment theory as applied to forensic settings.

Anne Aiyegbusi is Consultant Nurse and works in a forensic mental health service in West London. She has worked and led in the development of clinical nursing practice within a number of forensic settings in the UK. Anne is particularly interested in the nurse–patient relationship with people who have personality disorders and the clinical application of attachment theory. Anne is a member of the executive board of the International Association for Forensic Psychotherapy and is currently completing a PhD. She previously completed the Diploma in Forensic Psychotherapeutic Studies at the Portman Clinic.

Miranda Barber is currently employed by Herefordshire Primary Care Trust as Lead Clinical Psychologist for the Rehabilitation and Recovery Service, and is an honorary lecturer with the School of Forensic and Family Psychology at Birmingham University. One of her clinical interests lies in the importance of attachment theory in shaping and understanding the clinician–client relationship.

Sarita Bose is Senior Clinical Nurse and has worked at Broadmoor Hospital for the past 12 years. She has previously worked in the hospital's Centralised Groupwork Service as a nurse therapist, co-facilitating a range of psychological group therapies. Sarita has completed the Diploma in Forensic Psychotherapeutic Studies at the Portman Clinic and, more recently, an MSc in the Psychodynamics of Human Development at the British Association of Psychotherapists.

Valerie Anne Brown is Team Leader at Broadmoor Hospital, West London Mental NHS Trust.

Tom Clarke is a senior mental health nurse and researcher with a special interest in practice-led development and research.

Jenifer Clarke-Moore has worked as a nurse in forensic mental health services and services for people with personality disorders for many years. She has led in the delivery of psychodynamic nursing practice within forensic services and has also provided psychological therapies. Jenifer is currently working as Consultant Nurse with a specialist personality disorder service at Gwent Healthcare NHS Trust, Wales.

Katie Downes came to mental health nursing as a mature student, having worked for 13 years as a community health care assistant. The experience fuelled her interest in the psychological care of pain and distress. Ultimately this led to a desire to understand the trauma that invariably lies behind the collapse of mental stability. She has spent six years working in a service for women with severe personality disorders and is currently Acting Clinical Nurse Manager within a forensic setting caring for men with personality disorders and mental illness. The relationship between the child and their earliest significant carer(s) remains her greatest concern and she is indebted to the Tavistock Centre for the postgraduate training she received there.

Neil Gordon is a forensic psychotherapist and psychotherapy supervisor who project leads the English National Personality Disorder Development Programme (Knowledge and Understanding Frameworks). He works as a senior fellow in the Personality Disorder Institute in Nottingham where he delivers a range of educational programmes and is involved in research and service development activity. Neil was previously Consultant Nurse in the Personality Disorder Directorate at Rampton High Security Psychiatric Hospital.

Malcolm Kay is Group Analyst and Adult Psychotherapist at Royal Cornhill Hospital, Aberdeen. He originally trained as a registered mental nurse and has worked with forensic patients in inpatient and outpatient settings. He is indebted to his training on the Diploma in Forensic Psychotherapy at the Portman Clinic.

Amanda Lowdell is Clinical Nurse Specialist in psychodynamic psychotherapy at Ravenswood House Medium Secure Unit, Hampshire Partnership NHS Trust. She has previously worked as counsellor, psychotherapist, nurse therapist and supervisor for the prison service. Amanda has a special interest in the emotional impact on staff who work therapeutically with offenders in secure environments.

Stephen Mackie is Consultant Forensic Nurse Psychotherapist at the Portman Clinic, Tavistock and Portman NHS Foundation Trust. He is a member of the Lincoln Centre for Psychotherapy and is in private practice.

Maria McMillan began mental health nurse training at St Thomas and Guy's after studying and teaching music in London for several years. She qualified in 1996 and has taken further postgraduate studies at the Portman Clinic and the British Association of Psychotherapists. Maria lives and works in East London.

Suzanne McMillan is Service Manager in an acute mental health service in West London. Suzanne originally trained as a mental health nurse and has previously managed secure services for women, including services for women with personality disorders. Suzanne has a special interest in women's mental health.

Rebecca Neeld is Group Analyst and Lead Nurse at the Cassel Hospital. She has 20 years' experience of working in various therapeutic communities with people who have personality disorder.

Joanne Roberts has worked as Consultant Service User for HAFAL Cymru for approximately 14 years. She is a leading voice for service users in Wales, particularly for women service users and for those who are detained in secure services. Joanne has given expert verbal evidence to the Houses of Parliament and the Welsh Assembly Government on the proposed changes to the Mental Health Act 1983. She has addressed national conferences and continues to champion the rights of service users both locally and nationally.

Christopher Scanlon is Consultant Psychotherapist, South London & Maudsley NHS Trust (SLaM) and was formerly Consultant Psychotherapist and lead for Training and Consultation, Henderson Hospital Services until its closure. He has acted as a professional advisor to the Social Inclusion Unit, Department for Communities and Local Government; the training and human resource committee for Dangerous Severe Personality Disorder (DSPD) Project at the Home Office/Department of Health and was a member of the Department of Health Severe Personality Disorder, Expert Advisory Group making recommendations to NIMHE (2003) *Personality Disorder: No Longer a Diagnosis of Exclusion.* He is also Senior Visiting Research Fellow at the Centre for Psycho-social Studies, University of West England (UWE) and honorary senior lecturer in Forensic Mental Health, St George's University of London. He is also trustee of the Zito Trust – a major mental health charity campaigning for improved services for mentally disordered offenders and their victims.

Gillian Tuck is Practice Development Nurse at West London Mental Health Trust. She has worked in medium and high secure mental health services for the past seven years, specialising in the care of patients who have personality disorder. She has a particular interest in the psychodynamics of forensic mental health nursing as well as the use of a systems psychodynamic approach to examining organisations. Gillian has completed a Masters degree in 'Consultation and the organisation: Psychoanalytic approaches' at the Tavistock Clinic and University of East London.

Subject Index

Note: page numbers in *italics* refer to diagrams and information contained in tables.

Author Index